THE
MENOPAUSE
WEIGHT LOSS
SOLUTION

A Woman's Guide to Menopause
Without the Pounds

MICHELLE BITON

Author of *The Instant Anxiety Solution*

Hatherleigh Press, Ltd.

62545 State Highway 10

Hobart, NY 13788, USA

hatherleighpress.com

THE MENOPAUSE WEIGHT LOSS SOLUTION

Text Copyright © 2025 Michelle Biton, BodyMind Publications LLC

Library of Congress Cataloging-in-Publication Data is available.

ISBN: 978–1–961293–23–6

Printed in the United States

The authorized representative in the EU for product safety and
compliance is Catarina Astrom, Blästorpsvägen 14, 276 35 Borrby,
Sweden. info@hatherleighpress.com

10 9 8 7 6 5 4 3 2 1

PRAISE FOR *THE MENOPAUSE WEIGHT LOSS SOLUTION*

"Practical, inspiring, empowering…a must-read for every woman who is ready to make menopause a magnificent transition into healthy living."
   —**Beth Hedva, PhD,** *author of Embodied Awareness: An Introduction to Spiritually Directed Therapy*

"Michelle Biton's approach to menopause is groundbreaking and empowering. *The Menopause Weight Loss Solution* is not just a guide to navigating hormonal changes—it's a comprehensive blueprint for women looking to reclaim their vitality, confidence, and well-being."
   —**Lorne Brown,** *Clinical Director of Acubalance, host of Conscious Fertility Podcast*

"*The Menopause Weight Loss Solution* is a fantastic book with valuable information for every menopausal woman. As a celebrity trainer whose primary focus is strength training, I give Michelle a thumbs-up for doing a great job breaking down this complex subject."
   —**Ramona Braganza,** *celebrity fitness trainer*

CONTENTS

PREFACE

Menopause can be a bitch…if you let it.

I am currently going through perimenopause, and I am determined to do it WITHOUT extra pounds, feeling fat and ugly, or having issues like hot flashes, night sweats, depression, urine leakage or many of the other uncomfortable symptoms that women suffer.

Menopause is typically known to be the time when women are "past their prime," old, worn and unattractive. Accordingly, many relationships break up. Women get passed over for younger women.

But there is more to this story. And mindsets are changing.

This book is about breaking barriers, changing mindsets, mastering menopause *naturally* with the use of nutrition, exercise, nervous system manipulation, and stepping into your personal power.

This book is about *celebrating* your new stage of life…one of power, beauty, elegance, wisdom, radiance, sophistication, and *sexiness*.

This book is about *embracing* your new role of "self-fulness" and finding your well-deserved beauty, sexuality, and spirituality.

No more throwing in the towel! Menopause does *not* have to mean old, worn, overweight and unattractive.

This book is about *reclaiming* yourself, your beauty, your sexual power and your body.

Society is changing. 50-year-old women are the new 40s. Middle-aged women are playing sexy leading roles in movies, winning Oscars for leading roles, and posing naked, without makeup, displaying their beautiful, sexy figures after 50 (and being proud of it)!

Gone are the days of mourning our youth, our beauty, and reproductive losses. This new stage is a rite-of-passage.

Now we must learn to celebrate it, own it, and step into our new skin. YOU ARE BEAUTIFUL.

Let's kick menopause's ass!

—Michelle

INTRODUCTION

What do menopause and pregnancy have in common?

Pregnancy and menopause are both times of major hormonal, physical, mental, and emotional transitions in women's lives.

Both pregnancy and menopause come with a lot of fear, uncertainty, body changes, and hormones.

But, despite what common rhetoric tells us, we *do not* have to have painful, terrible, negative experiences. *No way.*

I am going to show you, just as I showed over one million pregnant women 20 years ago, how to master this major transition in your life.

Menopause does not have to be terrible. You absolutely can look great and beat many of the menopause-related symptoms.

If you think about it, how many women do you know that have had positive experiences during menopause?

I am almost certain that most of you do not know anyone who had a positive menopause experience because people love to share their horror stories and negative experiences. Very rarely do people talk about their positive experiences.

The same thing happened with pregnancy.

And so, I went on my way 20 years ago to change that belief that women must have rough pregnancies, gain tons of weight, and struggle to lose their baby-weight afterwards.

I wrote a hugely successful book called *Pregnancy Without Pounds* which helped over a million women around the world get through pregnancy looking and feeling fantastic and melting their pregnancy pounds in record time post-delivery.

There is no question that menopause is a transition—it is a huge change in your life. It is the end of one chapter and the beginning of another chapter. As with any transition, navigating blindly can lead to discouragement.

Top three mistakes most menopausal women make:

1. Believing that they are invisible, that they don't matter, that they don't have a voice.

2. Believing that they are past their prime. Thinking that their time has come and gone; that they are no longer beautiful; that they don't have a voice; they are not attractive; they are invisible.

3. Letting go of healthy "self-care" behaviors, including dressing up, putting on makeup, doing their hair, taking care of their figure, watching their calorie intake, etc.

Now I'm going to show you how to **master your menopause.**

I'm going to show you how to melt your menopause pounds and get through this major transition looking good and feeling great.

You are leaving behind the Reproductive stage and entering the Wise stage.

Be proud. Feel beautiful. You've EARNED it.

DISCLAIMER

The information in this book is for educational purposes only. This information is not to be treated as therapy nor medical advice. This book is a generalized program for the mass population. Please ask your doctor, nutritionist, therapist or trainer about concepts, supplements or exercises that you want to try in this book before acting. Your doctor, nutritionist, therapist, and trainer, know you and your situation best.

CHAPTER 1

THE S.H.R.I.N.K. FORMULA

N ow let's get started to learn the truth about how to get through menopause looking great and feeling fantastic, and how to avoid those painful and annoying symptoms, like weight gain, thick waist, hot flashes, night sweats, urine leakage, constipation and painful sex.

The average age for menopause is 45–55 years old, with the most common age of onset at 51 years. Perimenopause or pre-menopause typically lasts 2 to 8 years and is often the most difficult, as this is the time when many women experience all the nasty "menopausal" symptoms.

Interestingly, women who smoke or are underweight tend to have earlier menopause, while women who are overweight tend to have later onset. In general, women tend to have menopause around the same time their mother did.

Now we naturally go through many transitions in life that make us more susceptible to weight gain, and menopause is a major transition. But that doesn't mean you have to give in to it.

You absolutely can get through menopause without gaining 10, 20 or 30 pounds. There is a way to fight back. You can learn to work with your body (and not against it) to maintain a healthy body weight and appearance during menopause and that is what I am going to teach you with the S.H.R.I.N.K. formula.

What Exactly is Menopause?

Menopause is a natural process. You officially hit menopause when you do not get your period for 12 consecutive months. The ovaries stop making estrogen and progesterone and the period disappears. It signifies the end of the reproductive years and the beginning of the wise "goddess" years.

But that is the easy version. Menopause, or pre-menopause, can feel like a rollercoaster ride of hormones or a symphony of fireworks. The menstrual cycle becomes erratic, periods can become shorter or longer, sometimes lighter, other times heavier, with varying lengthens in between, and then just when you think you are finished, it comes back with a vengeance.

Perimenopause (or pre-menopause) is a transitional phase of menopause, and typically the time you feel the most difficult symptoms. This phase can start in your 30s or 40s and can last up to 10 years. You may notice mood changes, headaches, insomnia, body changes and many other symptoms.

At least 80 percent of women will experience menopausal symptoms of varying degrees and severity.

You might start to notice (sometimes even overnight):

- Slower metabolism
- Poor memory or brain fog

- Fat deposits increasing
- Weight gain around the middle (a.k.a. "menopause belly")
- Upper body thickening
- Flabby arms
- Sagging skin (especially around the neck, jawline and cheeks)
- Drooping breasts
- Thinning hair
- Increased facial hair
- Wrinkles and undereye bags
- Raging hormones
- Diminished eyesight
- Urinary tract infections
- Increased irritability and moodiness
- Difficulty sleeping (including falling asleep and staying asleep)
- Night sweats
- Hot flashes

- Increased anxiety

- Increased sadness

- Aching joints (wrists, shoulders, knees)

- Diminished sex drive

- Dry itchy skin

Navigating these body changes during perimenopause and menopause can be challenging, but the good news is they are solvable.

Menopause Weight Gain

Weight gain during menopause affects 65–70 percent of women. The average weight gain is 5–10 lbs.

A national health and nutrition survey discovered that **68 percent of women between ages 40 and 59 were classified as "overweight" or "obese."**

Factors such as genetics, hormones, metabolism, body type, lifestyle, even body weight pre-menopause all affect how much weight you will gain.

The good news is that losing just 5 percent of body weight can make a huge difference in your health.

Am I destined to have a flabby tummy forever?

Contrary to popular belief, you do not have to have a tummy problem for the rest of your life.

Due to reduced hormone production during menopause, often occurring in perimenopause, we naturally start losing muscle mass and increasing fat storage. Typically, we lose muscle mass around the midsection, and it is replaced with fatty tissue deposits, hence the menopause belly appearance. This physical change happens quickly.

Our genetics play a role, if you're mother had weight gain around her midsection after menopause, there is a high likelihood that you will too, unless you do something to prevent it.

The menopause belly, like any weight gain, does bring health issues like increased risk of diabetes, high blood pressure, breathing issues, heart disease, arthritic pain and more.

Focusing solely on weight loss will not fully combat menopause belly—it will only leave you with a smaller flabby stomach because you're not firming the muscles *below* the surface. What you need **is the right *combination* of specific muscle building exercises and fat loss to get your midsection back.**

Beware of Cortisol Levels

Cortisol is the body's primary stress hormone. It surges when we sense stress or danger.

Cortisol levels become elevated naturally as we age. Cortisol stimulates the liver to increase the production and release of blood sugar and helps the body convert fats, proteins, and carbohydrates to usable energy. **If you are stressed out all the time, you will deposit fat in your belly area.**

Ironically, intense exercise can also increase cortisol levels and fat storage. Yep, you read that right! But, if done correctly, moderate exercise and endorphins will suppress this high cortisol production and work in your favor. Just 20 minutes of exercise a day can help you to reduce your cortisol hormone to a manageable level.

Avoid the "Letting Go" Trap

During menopause, many women stop taking care of themselves, stop dressing up, working out, dying their hair, watching what they eat, and so on. I'm not saying that you should go out and get plastic surgery or spend every few weeks at the hairdresser. What I am saying is that neglecting care of yourself is a trap. That extra indulgence, piece of cake, bottle of wine, fancy desert, missed workout, canceled gym membership, and so on, will lead to gaining one pound, two pounds, three pounds…before you know it, you are 20 to 30 pounds overweight with grey hair and nothing to wear because none of your old clothes fit.

This common scenario feels terrible and takes a serious toll on your mental health. To prevent this scenario, you must continue to take care of yourself every day for you. Your mental health will be much better if you are feeling better about your situation.

If you feel better about yourself, you will take better care of yourself. You will attract more positive things in your life. Your mental health will be better. You will feel more positive about your life. Your relationships will be better.

Of course, you can absolutely have a bite of cheese-cake, a glass of wine, or a night out with the girls—just in moderation and with your eyes wide open.

Remember, it's a holistic approach. You can't eat your way out of exercise, and you can't exercise your way out of a poor diet. Stay healthy in your body, mind and spirit.

The S.H.R.I.N.K. formula was developed to give you the power to fight back against the negatives that come with menopause and to avoid the natural decline in health and beauty that comes with age. These six easy steps will help you cruise through menopause both looking good and feeling great.

Introducing the six-step formula to help you master your menopause: S. H. R. I. N. K.

1. **Stimulate** Your Metabolism

2. **Harness** the Power of Your Vagus Nerve

3. **Reinforce** the 8 Nutritional Strategies

4. **Incorporate** Daily Pelvic Floor & Core exercises

5. **Nurture** Mindfulness & Mindful Eating

6. **Know** Your Female Powers with Confidence

The S.H.R.I.N.K. formula will help you take charge of your menopause experience. The following chapters will discuss each aspect of the S.H.R.I.N.K. method so that as soon as you notice any menopause symptoms you can immediately fight back.

Be proactive and move fast. If you do not, you most likely will experience things like weight gain, "middle-tire syndrome," hot flashes, night sweats, memory issues, joint pain, urinary incontinence, a feeling of disconnect from your body, moodiness and many more annoying symptoms.

Wherever you are in your menopause journey, there is always room to make positive changes. Even if you take away just one **new positive thing to implement**, you are moving forward in mastering your menopause.

Chapter Takeaways

#1: Menopause is Natural and Can Be Positive

Menopause is the natural process that occurs for women between ages 45–55. It typically takes

7–10 years to complete and is the end of the reproductive years and beginning of the wise years. Perimenopause (before the period stops for 12 consecutive months) tends to be full of the difficult symptoms.

#2: The S.H.R.I.N.K. Formula

The six-step formula to help women master menopause and avoid all the common pitfalls and issues during menopause. A complete holistic program that incorporates body, mind and spirit.

#3: Avoid the Cortisol Trap

Cortisol is critical to understand during menopause, as it is the key to solving many menopause-related problems. If you avoid the **cortisol trap** and learn to work with the body rather than against it, you can accomplish not only better health and wellness, but better physical appearance as well.

CHAPTER 2

STIMULATE YOUR METABOLISM

As we age, our metabolism naturally declines. **Most women's metabolism drops by 10 percent each decade after 20 years old.**

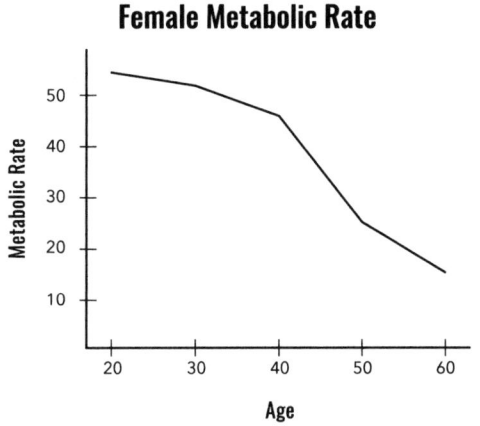

Female Metabolic Rate

The decrease in estrogen and progesterone, as well as natural aging, triggers metabolic changes in the body. From the age of 20, our declining metabolism affects our body weight, appearance, and energy level. To many women, it can feel like these changes happen overnight.

You might find that you are exercising and eating the same way as you always did, yet you are gaining weight, especially around your midsection.

In simple terms, metabolism is the **rate at which your body works**. During menopause, where you gain weight, and how much, will depend on a combination of your genetics, your body type, your lifestyle, your activity level, and your diet.

How fast or slow you gain or lose weight, your body shape, as well as the speed of your metabolism are determined by *which* metabolic type you fall under.

The S.H.R.I.N.K. formula takes this information into account and helps all female body types counter the natural side effects of menopause.

The reality is that during menopause weight gain will happen to all women and tend to distribute around the middle, certain body types will have an easier time than others both gaining and losing weight.

There are three main metabolic body types for women:

1. **Ectomorph:** long and lean

2. **Endomorph:** round

3. **Mesomorph:** muscular

The three metabolic body types are determined by your stature, shape and composition.

Female Metabolic Body Type Traits

Ectomorph

Ectomorphs are long and lean, and typically have a fast metabolism, making them naturally more skinny, bony, with low body fat. They tend to have smaller waists, narrow hips and shoulders, small joints and long arms and legs. Ectomorphs typically have a hard time gaining muscle and fat. They tend to like caffeine and other stimulants and usually prefer to eat protein over carbohydrates.

Endomorph

Endomorphs are the softer, rounder body type with a higher percentage of body fat. They typically have larger joints, a bigger body frame and slower metabolism. They typically carry their weight throughout their entire body. Their metabolism tends to be slower than the other two body types and, as a result, they tend to store fat easily and struggle to lose weight. They typically like carbs and sweets. The endomorph is the most common body type for women.

Mesomorph

Mesomorphs are naturally muscular with a tendency to gain muscle and strength easily. They tend to have a balanced physique and body composition with broad shoulders and medium-sized joints. They tend to have an efficient metabolism, good body tone, and respond to exercise well, however if they are not mindful, they can gain body fat around the midsection.

Basal Metabolic Rate

This is the number of calories burned at the basic life functioning level. **Your BMR accounts for 60-70 percent of the calories we use, burn or expend.** It includes the basic functions of breathing, circulation, nutrient production and heartrate.

Your BMR is influenced by age, weight, height, gender, environmental temperature, exercise, activity level, and diet. The goal is to increase your BMR. This will help you burn more calories throughout your day.

Weight Gain During Menopause

During menopause, a women's ability to burn calories gets cut by 30 percent or more. **By the time she reaches middle age, she will have to work almost twice as hard to burn the same about of calories as she did in her 20s.**

The average weight gain during menopause is **5–10 pounds,** but that is 10 pounds of fat weight! One pound of muscle *weighs the same* as one pound of fat, but **one pound of fat takes up *five times* the space as one pound**

of muscle. A pound of fat is bulky, fluffy, and about the size of a grapefruit. A pound of muscle is smaller, hard, and about the size of a tangerine.

You see the problem? **You gain size as you get older because of the body's natural composition changes.** Most of this volume comes from fat because it is five times bigger than muscle.

But the problem goes deeper. **The metabolic rate of muscle is three times more active than fat.** This means that muscle burns more calories than fat, even while your body is at rest. So not only do we naturally get bigger as we age, but our bodies physiologically slow down, meaning we must work **three times** as hard to burn the same number of calories than we did when we were younger.

This decrease in metabolic rate means you will burn roughly 200–250 calories less per day during menopause. Now if you multiply 250 per day out times 7 days a week, that equals 1,750 calories per week.

If you multiply 1,750 calories times 2, to account for a 2-week period, you will burn 3,500 calories. Now, I am the last person to advocate for calorie counting, but if you do the simple math, you can see how weight gain becomes a problem for menopausal women.

Why? Because **1 pound of fat is 3,500 calories**.

you see where I'm going with this...**every 2 weeks during menopause you will gain 1 pound of fat**—and that is just because of the body's naturally slowed down metabolism.

And if you calculate that rate over 5–10 years of menopause, you can see how easy it is for women to gain 5, 10, 15 or 20 pounds over menopause.

The Body Types During Menopause

Ectomorphs

Even though ectomorphs have less body fat and a faster metabolism than the other body types, during menopause they will likely experience some composition changes and fat storage in the abdominal area simply due to changing hormones and the natural slowing down of the metabolism. Ectomorphs typically have less muscle mass, which makes them more prone to reduced metabolism during menopause.

Endomorphs

During menopause, endomorphs will have a naturally higher body fat percentage and struggle with weight management more than the other body types. Endomorphs are prone to a slower metabolism, less lean muscle, and more overall body fat, and the further muscle reduction and slowing of the metabolism make weight gain even more of an issue during menopause. Weight gain tends to be all over the body, including around the midsection.

Mesomorphs

During menopause, mesomorphs will likely experience a shift in fat distribution with more fat deposits in the abdominal area. How much depends on diet, exercise and lifestyle. Mesomorphs typically maintain more lean muscle which helps to alleviate some of the menopausal weight gain and slower metabolism. Even with a naturally higher metabolism, mesomorphs will need to adjust their eating and exercise during menopause to encourage hormonal balance, good metabolism and a healthy body weight and appearance.

The Importance of Building Muscle

As we age, our muscle mass decreases. When we lose muscle mass, we **lose both our shape** and our **ability to burn calories efficiently.**

Building and maintaining muscle mass will stimulate your metabolism. The higher the percent of muscle on your body, the more calories you will burn and the slimmer and more toned you will appear. Building muscle mass is also important for building bone density, something that also decreases during menopause.

Now I'm not talking about becoming a body builder; what I am talking about is **building up some lean muscle mass by doing light weight-bearing exercises.** You don't even have to even go to the gym to do this.

Luckily, it only takes minor changes to kickstart your metabolism. Simple things like lifting your body weight against gravity does the job perfectly. You can do them anywhere; they are easy to do and very effective. This includes exercises like push-ups, triceps dips, lunges and squats. My personal favorite is walking lunges.

Whatever exercise you choose, the important thing is to **make sure your workout routine includes strength training or resistance work rather than just cardio**. Read the suggestions below and find the movements that work best for you!

Ectomorphs

Ectomorphs should take a balanced approach to exercise during menopause with an emphasis on building muscle to increase the metabolism, provide good muscle tone, minimize weight gain, and improve overall health and fitness. Concentrate on doing resistance training at the gym or on their own with their own body weight 2–3 times a week, in addition to regular cardiovascular exercise. Even though ectomorphs will gain the least amount of weight of the body types, they are not immune to having a menopause belly. Because they have a smaller frame, even small changes can be noticeable to them.

Endomorphs

Endomorphs should focus on minimizing weight gain and stimulating their metabolism during menopause. Focus on doing as much activity in your day as possible. The exercise strategy should focus on a balanced approach combining cardio and strength training. Focus on building lean muscle with higher repetitions, even do fun activities that involve doing cardio and using the whole body—like swimming, aquacise, Zumba dance class, aerobics, even pickleball.

Mesomorphs

Mesomorphs should focus on maintaining and/or building back their muscle mass so they can continue to have an efficient metabolism, good muscle tone, and minimize weight gain during menopause. Emphasize weightlifting or resistance training, 2–3 days a week, and regular cardiovascular activities 4–5 days a week. Focus on minimizing weight gain, boosting metabolism, and managing body fat.

What Kind of Resistance Training?

Resistance training can be done in several different ways. You can go to the gym and use the weight machines, use hand-held free weights, resistance bands, or simply use your **own body weight against gravity**.

Please note that it is critical to talk to your doctor *before* you do any exercises to make sure they are safe for you to do. The information in this book is for education only. It is of general nature and not specific to your situation. It is also important to perform each exercise properly to avoid injury and benefit from the exercises.

Good resistance training incorporates two types of exercises: **isotonic** and **isometric**.

Isotonic means working through the full range of motion. It involves muscle contractions where the muscle changes length and movement around a joint. Some examples of isotonic exercises are push-ups, lunges, and squats. Here are a few different lunges to try:

Lunges

1. Stand with your feet together

2. Step your right leg forward (big step)

3. Dip down to the floor and back up again, keeping your right knee directly over your right ankle)

4. Repeat up and down 12–15 times then switch to the other leg.

Alternating Lunges

1. Stand with your feet together

2. Step your right leg forward into a lunge (big step), and then push back up again to a standing position where both legs are back together.

3. Change legs and do the same thing on the other side, down and then back up to a standing position, alternating one leg at a time.

4. Make sure to keep your front knee directly over your ankle (do not let your knee extend further out than your front toes).

Isometric means contracting your muscles without changing their length or moving the surrounding joints. It involves holding a position for an extended period of time. The plank, for example, is a great isometric exercise. Other great isometric exercises are wall sits and static lunges.

Plank

1. Kneel on the floor and place your forearms on the ground in front of you with your palms down.

2. Tuck your bum under, into a pelvic tilt; only your forearms and knees (or toes if you more advanced) should be touching the ground.

3. Your body should form a line—do *not* stick your bum up in the air; instead, tuck your pelvis under to engage your abdominal muscles.

4. You should feel this exercise in your abs as well as your arms and legs, but not in your lower back! Hold for as long as you are able, working up to one minute.

You can challenge yourself by increasing the length of your hold, or by doing it from your toes instead of your knees. Remember to progress slowly—it's not a competition!

Other great exercises to try are:

- Push-ups (flat or incline, from knees or toes)
- Squats or jump squats
- Walking lunges
- Triceps dips
- Step ups
- Burpees

Intensity and Progressive Overload

Walking is low-impact, easily accessible, non-intimidating (unlike the gym), relatively easy on the joints, good for stress management and enjoyable. It's also an easy way to get outdoors, benefit from nature therapy, and may include a social aspect which are all important for mental health.

Many benefits of exercise are found at the **moderate intensity** levels. This means going for a **brisk walk** is an excellent choice for exercise (and my personal favorite).

In fact, going for a long, brisk walk is a great way to burn fat and avoid increasing your cortisol levels, which causes increased fat storage during menopause, and strengthens your emotional well-being.

Walking daily has many health benefits; it will improve cardiovascular health, balance and coordination; strengthen bones and muscles; improve mood, memory, and sleep; aid in managing blood pressure and diabetes; strengthen the immune system; and help you to lose weight.

To get even more *benefits* from walking you can increase the **intensity** and **duration** of your walk whenever you are ready. In other words, you can get more out of your "workout" simply by walking **faster** or walking for **longer**. You can even **add a hill** or two to your route, or speed walk or light jog for one block and then back to your regular pace for the next block and so on. This is the **Principle of Progressive Overload**, where you gradually increase the demands placed on the body to continue to make gains in muscle strength, endurance and overall fitness level. To stimulate muscle growth and fitness level, you need to progressively challenge your muscles by increasing their workload.

Another way this progression can be achieved is by implementing **interval training.** Interval training is the concept of adding in **short intervals of more intense exercise** to your workout to get your heart rate up and get you in better shape faster. For example, to increase the intensity of my walking workout, I either 1) head for the hills or a steady incline or 2) increase the *pace* of my walk, 3) add speed walking or light jog interval every few blocks, or 4) walk for *longer*, preferably one hour. You will be amazed at how your fitness level and endurance will quickly improve when you add a jog, a hill, or speed walk to your daily walk.

Be mindful of your body as you walk. Notice how it feels, paying special attention to your breathing, your blood circulating, your heart rate rising. Notice the environment around you, the sky, the landscape, and the terrain. Breath in the air. Concentrate on lengthening and deepening your breaths.

Applying the Principle of Progressive Overload

Aim for the hills or increase your pace or the length of your walk when you feel ready. **The optimal goal is to do 20–60 minutes of walking activity 5–7 days a week.** Focus on being active as often as you can—aim for using the stairs (instead of the elevator), walking to the store (instead of driving), dancing around the house (instead of sitting at the TV), even taking the dog for an extra walk or two around the neighborhood.

The goal is to reach 10,000 steps in a day. This is why tracking your steps can be such a great motivator. You can put on a pedometer or use a phone app to track how many steps you take per day. Pedometers are designed to count the number of steps a person takes, as opposed to the number of miles walked.

I know it may seem like a lot at first, but a simple paradigm shift around exercise is all that is needed. Exercise does not have to be hard work—in fact, it can be the opposite. Focus on gradually increasing the number of steps you take every day. You will be amazed at how fast your steps add up.

Walking is even a great way to solve problems. Working through problems when you are outside walking will allow you to naturally de-stress and calm the nervous system down, and be more "available" to solve problems. Give it a try, even if you don't have anyone to talk to, you can think through your problems when you are walking outside—you will be amazed at the clarity and grounding a walk will do for you!

You will see a huge difference in how you look and feel if you simply focus on doing more activity during your *entire* day.

Cardio

The most natural way to change your brain chemistry is with exercise. **Exercise releases endorphins and other neurochemicals which help improve our mood and give us a heightened sense of well-being**. When we exercise, the body gets flooded with an increase in serotonin, dopamine, and norepinephrine. **Serotonin** is responsible for feelings of serenity and hopefulness. **Dopamine** and **norepinephrine** are responsible for feelings of relaxation and happiness.

Both exercise and happiness increase antibody production in the body which builds immunity, meaning that we will not get sick as often.

In addition to your walking routine mentioned above, or instead, you can add some form of cardio a minimum of 3–5 times a week for 30–60 minutes at an intensity level of 60–75 percent of your maximum heart rate or a 6–7. 5 (maybe 8 when walking up hills) on your PRE (Perceived Rate of Exertion) scale.

Perceived Rate of Exertion (PRE) is a great, extremely simple way to measure your heart rate. It gets you to determine how hard you "feel" you are working on a scale of 0–10. 0=rest, 10=exercising very hard, like sprinting. Interestingly, your "feeling" of how hard you are working is very close to how hard you are actually working. Aim to exercise between a 6–7.5 or 8 on the PRE scale.

NOTE: If you choose walking to be your cardio, that is great. Just make sure to walk fast enough to get a moderate workout.

Other great cardio exercises include:

- Cycling (or using a recumbent bicycle)
- Deep water running

- Swimming

- Jogging (even walk/jog mix)

- Hiking

- Stair climbing

- Rowing

- Aerobics

- Walking

The Intense Exercise Paradox

When you were younger, the harder you worked out, the more fat you burned. But this is *not* the case during menopause.

Exercise helps us regulate our blood sugar levels and fat storage. It improves body density and increases the production of the "feel-good" neurotransmitter, serotonin, to improve our mood.

But we must be mindful of the fact that exercise during menopause is a double-edged sword. Exercise can create stress on the body, increasing our cortisol levels and increasing our potential for weight gain.

For example, an extra 30-minute push on the elliptical can actually *increase* our already spiked cortisol levels, causing us to store more fat. **Ironically, the increased cortisol levels will also cause us to eat more high-fat, salty foods,** which our body has a harder time burning off.

This increase in cravings for "comfort foods," which are typically high in fat and sugar, lead to more weight gain. Cortisol also has an intricate relationship with insulin, the hormone which controls our blood sugar.

During menopause, we must take a ***moderate approach*** to working out. Aim for a moderate intensity exercise to increase your metabolism, as this does not result in significant increases in cortisol levels.

Protein and Metabolism

One of the easiest ways to boost your metabolism is to add protein to every meal and snack. Protein produces the **highest thermic effect from food**, which is the amount of energy it takes to digest, absorb, and utilize the food, and thus increases your metabolic rate by 30 percent. In other words, your body takes more time to digest protein than fat or carbs, so you end up feeling **fuller for longer**.

For easy ways to increase your protein intake, try adding chicken breast or chickpeas to salad, low-fat cottage cheese to peaches, salmon to grilled vegetables, or chicken breast to stir-fry. Other good ways to increase the thermic effect of your food is by adding green tea, or spices like black pepper, chili powder, cayenne pepper, and ginger.

Essential Fatty Acids and Metabolism

The stomach and mind are strongly interconnected. The gut contains over 300 million neurons and affects our mood and behavior.

Research shows that eating the right kind of fat, in the right quantities, can help increase energy, speed up our metabolism, and alleviate anxiety and depression. Linoleic fatty acids (omega-3) and linolenic fatty acids (omega-6) are required to sustain life. Since the body cannot make them, however, they must be found in the diet.

Essential fats increase the efficient delivery of oxygen and nutrients to the tissues by increasing the flexibility of the red blood cell membranes and making the insides of arteries more slippery. These good fats increase the production of hemoglobin, which also increases the amount of oxygen available to cells—an essential factor in all energy functions.

Essential fats also optimize thyroid, adrenal, and other glandular functions. This leads to an increase in metabolic rate, which means that we burn more calories, even when sleeping. Some essential fats increase the activity of genes that manufacture the enzymes needed for fat burning and thermogenesis (body heat). Essential fats also suppress the appetite and decrease cravings for junk food by satisfying the body's need for fat.

Aim to eat things in moderation like:

- Avocado
- Fish
- Eggs
- Nuts
- Seeds
- Olive oil
- Flax oil

Chapter Takeaways

#1: The Nasty Truth about Metabolism

A woman's metabolism slows consistently as she gets older, at a rate of 10 percent each decade, after the age of 20 years old. **Decreased metabolism directly affects weight gain and increased fat storage.** Luckily there *are* concrete things you can do to fight back. Small changes can make a positive difference in your metabolic rate.

#2: Build Your Muscles Up

Building up lean tissue is very important in fighting back against a slowing metabolism. Muscle makes the body look firmer and work more efficiently overall, helping to reduce the effects of aging. Aim for lifting weights, using resistance tubing or dumbbells, or my favorite, using your own body weight against gravity.

#3: Add Protein to Every Meal

Adding protein to meals is *key* to looking and feeling great during menopause. It helps you balance out your portions, decrease overeating, increase satiety, and *boost* your metabolism. **Aim for a fist size of low-fat, high-quality protein at each meal.**

#4: Walk Your Weight Off

During menopause, walking is a great way to lose weight. Sounds too good to be true, but because doing too much intense exercise during menopause is counter-productive to weight loss, you want to do more moderate exercise. **Regular physical activity, versus doing one intense working on the weekend, will be more beneficial at increasing your metabolism long-term.** Aim for the hill, increase your pace, walk for longer, even walk and talk to work out your problem or increase your social connections—all great strategies to add more walking into your day.

CHAPTER 3

HARNESS THE POWER OF YOUR VAGUS NERVE

The same hormones that control your menstrual cycle also influence serotonin, the chemical in your brain that promotes feelings of well-being and happiness. **When estrogen levels drop during menopause, serotonin levels also fall.**

Reduced serotonin causes feelings of:

- Irritability
- Anxiety
- Unhappiness

- Dissatisfaction

- Frustration

- Anger

- Apathy

- Loss of pleasure in things you once enjoyed

- No longer enjoying relationships

- Difficulty falling asleep and staying asleep

- Difficulty feeling well rested

The best way to deal with hormonal changes during menopause is to employ excellent stress management strategies. Learning how to take charge of your nervous system is step #2 in the S.H.R.I.N.K. formula, and critical in helping you take charge of your menopause.

The parasympathetic nervous system (PSNS), also known as the rest-and-digest system, is responsible for helping you calm down, handle stress better, regulate your mood, and feel more relaxed, connected, and compassionate. **The PSNS is crucial to how we develop resilience and emotional well-being**, and is also responsible for things like creativity, acting mindfully, complex decision making, and the ability to feel love and have orgasms.

When we are stressed or anxious, the sympathetic nervous system (SNS) is activated, causes us to enter fight-or-flight mode. The amygdala releases stress hormones that cause your heart rate, breath rate, and blood pressure to rise, preparing you to be able to run, fight or hid to get you out of a dangerous situation (if needed). The stress and anxiety of modern life, and many other situations, cause our sympathetic nervous system to activate.

During menopause it is common to feel stressed and overwhelmed, not to mention disconnected, irritable, worried, anxious, depressed and questioning a lot of things in life.

If you're having a hard time regulating your emotions, feeling overwhelmed, or overly emotional, it's a good idea to activate your PSNS right away.

Getting to a **parasympathetic state** quickly and regularly is a key component of the S.H.R.I.N.K. formula. The more time you spend here, the easier it will be to get through all of menopause's hormonal challenges.

Knowing how to activate your parasympathetic nervous system on demand is something like having a superpower. Think of it as if you are hijacking your nervous system, being able to take you out of the stressful sympathetic state and into the calm, parasympathetic state, in seconds. The faster you can do this, the better it will be for you—body and mind.

You could think of it this way: the SNS acts as the gas in the car, while the PSNS acts like the brakes. **The PSNS slows the car down (a.k.a. your body and mind) to a safe speed.**

Activating the PSNS will help your body quickly recover from the intense emotional state of fight-or-flight mode. It will immediately slow the heart rate, breathing and blood pressure down and relax the whole body.

When the PSNS is activated, the amygdala quiets down and the prefrontal cortex is engaged so that we can think logically again, feel and sense of calm and grounding, and problem solve effectively. The ability to digest food also returns—it gets shut off during the fight-or-flight mode.

The goal is to learn how to shift the physiological sensations of the body on demand without harming yourself.

The Magic of the Vagus Nerve

The vagus nerve is your key to activating the PSNS. By stimulating the vagus nerve, we can activate the PSNS and achieve many health benefits.

A healthy parasympathetic response, governed by the vagus nerve, is essential for our emotional well-being and physical health.

The vagus nerve is the main nerve of the PSNS responsible for calming the body down after a stressful event. It consists of two bundles of nerves that run from the brain stem down the sides of the neck to the internal organs. It helps to control digestion, heart rate, voice, mood and the immune system.

By increasing your understanding of the vagus nerve, you will learn how to work with your nervous system, rather than getting trapped by it.

When the vagus nerve is activated, you will automatically take a deep sigh, breath or yawn. Personally, I feel my chest expand and my breathing deepens. When the breathing and heart rate slow down, you'll begin to feel more relaxed.

However, the vagus nerve can be damaged or even dysfunctional. When this is the case, the vagus nerve cannot do its job properly; in other words, it cannot calm you down effectively, leading you to feel physically, mentally and emotionally depleted. **The body will remain in an alert state of high stress.**

The pressures and stresses of modern life also tax our vagus nerve and parasympathetic nervous system leaving us in a state of high anxiety, depression and panic much of the time, all symptoms of a dysregulated nervous system.

The goal is to build your own "tool kit" of ways to activate your vagus nerve and calm yourself down when you need it most. You will find that certain strategies work best for you. It is important to find a few effective ways to activate your own PSNS in order to relax *on demand* and calm down when needed. Unfortunately, there is not a one size fits all solution. You have to discover which strategies work for you.

There are certain techniques that work best when you're feeling really anxious, while others are more effective when you're feeling only a little anxious.

For example, my favorite strategies when I get really stressed out include sprinting down the block or taking a freezing cold shower, but these may not sound appealing to you. My go-to-solution when feeling moderately stressed is pulling my ear back—it instantly hacks my nervous system and calms me down.

In general, **the more you do your exercises and activate your vagus nerve, the healthier you will be.**

Like going to the gym and training your bicep muscles, you can train your vagus nerve. The more "fit" you are, the quicker you will be able to activate your vagus nerve and your PSNS and de-stress.

You may find that you practice some of these techniques intuitively already. For the longest time, I didn't realize that I was activating my vagus nerve every time I walked my dog, which is something I love to do. Every time I stepped out the door, I would put a piece of peppermint gum in my mouth and do the "spaced out" eye gaze before walking. This immediately calmed me down. Now I know why! I was using four strategies to activate my vagus nerve at once: 1) chewing gum, 2) stimulating my taste, 3) doing a sight exercise, and 4) getting out in nature.

Practicing techniques that stimulate the vagus nerve regularly will increase your vagal tone. The higher your vagal tone, the healthier you will be.

High vagal tone leads to:

- Having a high tolerance for stress
- Having a high capacity for change
- Being able to push through challenges easily
- Having good self-regulation
- Being able to bounce back from stress quickly
- Being able to handle life's ups and downs
- Being resilient, flexible and open minded
- Being present, grounded and engaged in life

Low vagal tone leads to...

- Having a poor tolerance for stress
- Having a low capacity for change
- Having poor self-regulation
- Getting knocked off course easily
- Having an inflexible and rigid personality
- Becoming dysregulated easily
- Having a difficult time bouncing back from stress
- Having a hard time relaxing and recharging

Strategies to Activate Your Vagus Nerve

Cold Exposure

Cold exposure is a great way to quickly activate your PSNS. Aim to find something quick and very cold to "surprise" your system and distract your mind. Make sure that you can endure it long enough to feel that "shock" or "surprise," but not too long that you will hurt yourself.

Researchers have found that regular cold exposure helps to lower the SNS fight-or-flight response and increase the PSNS activity through the vagus nerve.

Here are some great cold techniques that work wonders in helping to activate the vagus nerve's calming effects:

- Splashing icy water on your face several times.
- Taking a freezing cold shower.
- Submerging your face in cold water.

- Putting a cold pack on your cheek or back of your neck.

- Putting your hand in a bucket of ice water.

Burst of Exercise

When you are feeling very anxious, a quick burst of intense exercise can work wonders.

A burst of intense exercise requires 100 percent focus and attention, distracting the mind from the stressful event. During the burst of exercise, the sympathetic nervous system becomes dominant, causing an increase in breathing, heart rate, and the release of stress hormones.

After the exercise finishes, the parasympathetic nervous system becomes dominant, bringing the body back to a state of homeostasis and balance. This recovery period, slows the body down returning the heart rate, breathing and stress hormones to normal levels. This helps to lower stress and promote an overall calming effect.

Now both body and mind feel rejuvenated.

Here are a few ideas:

- Sprint to the end of the block.

- Do push ups until you reach exhaustion.

- Do jumping jacks, knee raises, or burpees until you reach exhaustion.

- Run on the spot, bringing your knees up high to hit your hands, alternating legs, as many times as you can.

If you're only a little stressed rather than extremely, focus on doing low to moderate aerobic exercise that you enjoy for a similarly positive effect on your PSNS.

- Go for a swim.

- Go for a bike ride.

- Head to the hills for a hike.

- Go for a brisk walk.

Exercise has been shown to increase *vagal tone*, which decreases your anxiety naturally.

Singing or Humming

The vagus nerve surrounds your voice box, or larynx. This means that humming and singing are excellent ways to stimulate your vagus nerve and de-stress your body and mind. The vibrations massage the section of your vagus nerve near your vocal cords, activating the PSNS and telling your body that it is safe.

Hop in the car, shower, or wherever you feel comfortable, and sing loud and proud! It doesn't matter what you sound like; singing loudly will activate your vagus nerve and help you feel much more relaxed.

Visualization

Visualization and imagery activate the PSNS.

Picture yourself in "your happy place," a place you love. Try to take it even further and "hear the sounds of the waves," "feel the wind through your hair," and "the scent of the flowers in the air." Adding pleasure will further activate the PSNS.

Similarly, saying a mantra to yourself can work to calm you down and activate your PSNS. I personally use mantras all the time to coach myself. They're a very good way to engage your wandering mind and provide you with a sense of safety by grounding you.

Deep Breathing

A deep sigh is your body's natural way to reset your nervous system and release tension from the body.

Typically, we inhale about 12–14 times a minute. Practice slowing your breathing down to 6 or 7 times a minute to reduce stress and anxiety. Concentrate on breathing deeply into your diaphragm and expanding with deep inhales and slow, long exhales. This will help to reduce your body's fight-or-flight response to stress and can have a profound impact in reducing emotional pain.

"Silent Screaming"

Anxiety, fear, guilt, shame—whatever it is you're feeling, try letting it out with a good silent scream. Screaming releases negative emotions and stress by activating the vagus nerve.

Take a deep breath in and then let it out with a big silent scream, a scream into a pillow, or even a real scream (if appropriate). You will feel much better afterwards.

A Good Belly Laugh

We always knew that laughing was good for us, did you know that it actually activates your PSNS by stimulating your diaphragm, and thereby triggering a physiological relaxation response?

Yes, by allowing yourself to laugh, you can activate your vagus nerve on demand, taking control of your body and your mood.

Cry Your Feelings Out

Crying is another great way to activate your PSNS and calm both your mind and body down quickly. It will restore emotional balance and dull pain allowing you to get to the other side of your "issue" and move forward.

Feeling your emotion is the only way to get to the other side and reduce your emotional suffering. When we avoid our emotions, it only makes the problem get bigger.

Nature Therapy

Nature therapy, or immersing yourself in nature, lowers cortisol levels and blood pressure in as little as 15 minutes.

Walking in the nature is a great way to activate your parasympathetic nervous system and calm down quickly and *naturally* from stress. To me, walking in the trees, listening to the birds, is like my meditation. I use this time to problem solve, process things and ground myself.

Apply Lip Balm

This is one of my favorite go-to things that I do throughout the day. I love to apply and re-apply my favorite natural lip balm.

Did you know that your lips are 100 times more sensitive than your fingertips?

Your lips are the most sensitive part of your body and have over 1 million nerve endings that, once activated, will help trigger the PSNS's rest-and-relax response?

Something so easy is very effective at calming you down.

Gargle Loudly

Gargling water, believe it or not, can help activate your vagus nerve and allow your body to relax and calm down.

Gargling, like singing, mechanically stimulates the vagal nerve by vibrating the nerve fibers in the back of the throat.

Cuddling

Cuddling a pet or someone you love releases serotonin, dopamine, and oxytocin.

Pets really are therapeutic and can help reduce stress and stimulate "happy" hormones. This is my top "feel good" technique.

The Pencil Technique

My go-to favorite technique when I'm feeling anxious, down or upset is to put a pencil lengthwise between my teeth. This exercise will trick your mind into believing you are happy, it will release "happy" chemicals, and help you to instantly feel better.

Give it a try. Look in the mirror, doesn't it look like your mouth is smiling with that pencil between your teeth? Believe it, you *will* feel better if you try this. I do this exercise all the time when I am stressed out or having an off day!

Progressive Muscle Relaxation

Progressive muscle relaxation is a self-help deep muscle relaxation technique. It is a great way to deal with the stress and anxiety of the fight or flight response of the sympathetic nervous system.

The technique involves tensing a group of muscles, holding, and then relaxing the muscles. The idea is to put your mind in your muscle, tensing and relaxing each muscle group separately, working from the top of your body down or vice versa.

For example, focus on the muscles in your calves, tighten the muscles as much as you can for five seconds, then let go of the tension and let the muscles relax. Work your way up your body to your thighs, glutes, abdomen, back, shoulders, arms, and so on, one area at a time.

The idea is that the muscles will become more relaxed than they were before you started the exercise. Relaxed muscles require less oxygen, which allows your breathing and heart rate to slow down and you to feel calmer.

This is a great mind-body technique. Muscle relaxation leads to mental calmness. The more time you spend in a parasympathetic state, the healthier you will be both mentally and physically.

Activate Your Senses

Another great strategy to activate your PSNS is to "wake up" your senses. We have our 5 regular senses: touch, taste, sight, smell, hearing. I like to add a sixth sense to the list: proprioception.

Proprioception is your body's ability to know where it is in space. If someone's proprioception sense is weak, they will likely be clumsy, trip and fall a lot, bump into things frequently and not know how hard or soft to squeeze something.

The more we activate and engage our six senses, the quicker it will get us to our calm, relaxed, and happy state, and the healthier we will feel, so practice them daily.

Sight

Look at your favorite picture, watch your favorite movie, go to your favorite location, whatever you can do to look at something pleasurable to help you take a deep "ahh" breath.

Smell

Light a candle, smell flowers or a favorite scent, smell your favorite meal or desert, whatever you can do to trigger that "ahh" moment.

Hearing

Listen to the sound of the ocean or rain falling, play your favorite songs, talk to a friend on the phone, whatever you can do to hear something pleasurable.

Taste

Eat your favorite food, chew your favorite gum, or suck on your favorite candy to get that pleasurable taste.

Touch

Go for a relaxing massage, get a mani/pedi, hug your dog (my favorite), or whatever you can do to activate your sense of touch.

Proprioception

Use a weighted blanket or vest, put on ankle weights, get a deep pressure massage, get/give a strong bear hug.

Chapter Takeaways

#1: Get to a Parasympathetic State

Aim to spend most of your time in the parasympathetic state. This will help you manage of the fluctuating hormones, moodiness, emotional instability, stress, and anxiety during menopause. Being able to hijack your nervous system on demand and quickly change your emotional response, gives you an incredible sense of power and confidence. The more time you spend in a parasympathetic state, the healthier and happier you will be.

#2: Activate Your Vagus Nerve

The vagus nerve is your superpower. It is the way to quickly activate the PSNS and change your emotional reaction. **Aim for high vagal tone, as this will build up your emotional resilience and allow you to handle stress better.** You'll be amazed to find that things which used to bother you simply don't anymore.

#3: Build Your Toolkit

Menopause can be an emotional rollercoaster, so **build your toolkit of technique so you can hack your own nervous system and calm down quickly**. Having these strategies in place *before* you need them is critical in being able stay on top of your emotional health.

CHAPTER 4

REINFORCE THE EIGHT NUTRITIONAL STRATEGIES

Nutrition is step #3 in the S.H.R.I.N.K. formula. To learn how to counter the negative effects of aging, it's important to eat the *right* foods. It's important to avoid going "on" and "off" this plan. It is designed to be a lifestyle. Dieting is only a temporary solution that will in the end up with poor results and increased fat storage.

Diets can temporarily work, but ultimately set us up for failure. In fact, **only 5 percent of people who lose**

weight from dieting successfully keeping their weight off long-term.

The other 95 percent continue the struggle, going on diet after diet. Instead, it is critical to create a routine that is **moderate** so you can **maintain your success long-term**.

Avoid Cutting Carbs

A lot of women believe that, if it's not a lack of exercise causing menopausal weight gain, then it *must* be the carbs. Carbs become evil. It's so easy to think that, if we just cut out pasta, bread, and bagels, then we'll surely shed the stubborn weight.

Despite all the voices telling us that ditching carbs is the magic solution to all weight gain problems, **for women over 40, avoiding carbohydrates is actually a mistake.**

I'm not talking about carbs like white bread, pasta, pastries, cake, chips, deserts. Cutting back the junk food, simple carbs, white sugar and processed foods will certainly help with weight loss and improving your overall health. I'm talking about healthy carbs like whole grains, brown rice, oats, barley, millet, quinoa, wheat, and rye. These foods add lots of fibre and nutrients, and increase digestion time, which helps to reduce overall calorie consumption.

Personally, if I'm trying to drop a few pounds, I eat lots of vegetables with protein, like a salmon salad or chicken stir-fry. I might add a sweet potato, yam, or brown rice at times.

Unfortunately, cutting carbs and focusing on diet alone is not enough to get rid of stubborn menopause fat. This is because **mid-life weight gain has very little to do with exercise or diet.**

We must take a holistic approach and look at the whole picture.

What Actually Happens During Menopause?

The combination of increased cortisol, reduced hormones, slower metabolism, reduced muscle mass, and weak abdominal muscles all contribute to the menopause belly and stubborn weight loss.

But there is another factor that affects weight gain during menopause…our **satiety level.**

Satiety in simple terms is the feeling of being sated or full. It is the physical and psychological "satisfaction" that someone feels after a meal. Someone can have either **high satiety** or **low satiety**. With "low satiety," the person will have the *inability* to know when they are full and keep eating. Someone with "high satiety" will know when they've eaten enough and feel satisfied to stop eating.

Due to changing hormone levels in menopause, our ability to feel "full" or "satisfied" from our meals *decreases*, causing us to eat *extra unnecessary calories*, resulting in weight gain.

Menopause, Hormones and Appetite

Estrogen: Decreasing estrogen levels during menopause *reduce* the hormones' ability to inhibit appetite, resulting in *increased appetite*.

Leptin: Decreasing leptin levels during menopause cause *reduce* feelings of fullness.

Ghrelin: Increasing ghrelin levels during menopause cause *increased* feelings of hunger.

Cortisol: Increasing levels of cortisol during menopause cause *increased* overeating.

Someone with low satiety will eat at least 10 percent more calories than someone with normal satiety. People with low satiety typically eat **larger portions, higher calories, higher fat** and **higher sugar foods** than someone with high satiety. They will also keep going back for more food when eating, resulting in **unnecessary weight gain**.

To avoid this and other natural weight gain traps, you must be proactive and fight back.

Your Eight Nutritional Strategies

#1: Boost Your Satiety

- **Eat protein with every meal.** This will help reduce your appetite, feel full faster and stay full for longer. Consuming protein slows digestion and increases the production of satiety hormones that stimulate *fullness* and *meal satisfaction*. Protein consumption also *reduces* the hormone ghrelin, which is your hunger hormone causing you to eat less.

- **Start with a broth-based soup or side salad before your meal** to fill up and curb your appetite.

- **Increase your fiber-rich foods to decrease hunger and increase satisfaction.** Fiber-rich foods add bulk to your meal, that causes you to take a longer time to digest your food and decrease your appetite.

- **Add fruit and grilled veggies to your meal to add a pop of color and taste.** This helps to increase satiety. Try things like watermelon, fresh berries, dried cranberries, grilled asparagus, or peaches to your meal.

- **Add a small handful of nuts to your salad to jazz it up and add some flavor.** This will help you feel more satisfied from your salad and eat less. Adding a small amount of healthy fats to your meal will also help you feel full for longer.

- **Add Brussels sprouts to your meal.** They are a high satiety food, high in fiber and water content, low in calories, nutrient dense, and they pack a powerful punch to a meal.

- **Add spices to your food.** This will help to increase meal satisfaction and decrease appetite.

- **Put your food on a smaller plate.** Fill it up and make it look appealing; smaller portions look bigger when framed by a small plate, tricking your mind into thinking that you are eating more.

- **Add a dash of olive oil or coconut oil, fresh avocado or a few of your favorite nuts to your meal.** Fats take longer to digest than carbohydrates and proteins, which slows digestion down helping you to feel full for longer.

Incorporate high-satiety foods like:

- Chicken breast, wild salmon or lean beef (preferably organic)
- Beans and legumes (black or kidney beans, chickpeas, lentils, split peas)
- Whole grains (quinoa, brown rice, barley, oats)
- Eggs
- Plain Greek yogurt
- Cottage cheese (low-fat)
- Tofu
- Baked potato with skin
- Edamame
- Apples
- Almonds
- Nuts (a few almonds, walnuts or cashews)
- Avocado
- Root vegetables (sweet potatoes, winter squash, carrots)
- Seeds (flax, hemp, chia)

#2: Load up on
High-Water Content Foods

High-water content foods are foods that have a lot of water in them, like fruits and vegetables, so they have volume without the calories.

Did you know?

- Fruit and vegetables contain over 90% water

- Broths and soups contain roughly 90% water

- Skim milk contains roughly 90% water

- Plain yogurt contains roughly 88% water

- Cottage cheese contains roughly 80% water

- Pasta, legumes, salmon, chicken breast contains 60–69% water

High-water content foods not only fill our stomachs up fast, they prevent us from consuming excess calories and help us lose weight.

Roughly 20 percent of the water we consume is through our food. The more high-water content foods you eat, the better. It will help your hydration level, help your joints feel better, help your digestive system, regulate your body temperature (which we *all* need during menopause), reduce your bloating, increase your energy, and help to flush toxins from your body.

Foods such as berries, melons and peaches are wonderful little treats that you can add to your salads and meals for a little extra color, flavor, bulk and excitement.

Great high-water content foods include:

- Melons (watermelon, cantaloupe, honeydew, casaba melon)
- Berries (strawberries, blueberries, raspberries, blackberries)
- Grapes
- Pineapple
- Peaches
- Oranges
- Cucumbers
- Lettuce
- Kale

- Zucchini

- Tomatoes

- Broccoli

- Bell peppers

- Celery

- Grapefruit

- Cabbage

- Spinach

- Pickles

Another great high-water content food strategy is to start your meal with a bowl of soup broth or green salad. This will help fill you up *before* your main course so that you will eat fewer calories with your overall meal. This is a fantastic strategy for weight loss and calorie reduction.

Great things to do with high-water content foods include:

- Make a fruit smoothie.

- Add berries as a salad topper.

- Add peaches, berries, or orange slices as a side accent.

- Make a fruit salad with a dollop of yogurt.

- Make fruit kabobs.

- Grill your fruit and veggies (pineapple, peaches, tomatoes, zucchini, broccolini are some that work especially well).

- Have veggies and dip (instead of chips and dip); some of my favorites for this are cucumbers, zucchini, carrots, cherry tomatoes, broccoli, peppers.

- Snack on frozen grapes or blueberries.

#3: Increase Daily Probiotic and Prebiotic Foods

Probiotics are critical for good health, digestion, a balanced mood, and the elimination of bloating. They control junk food cravings, blood sugar fluctuations, depression, anxiety, and weight gain.

An unhealthy gut has a hard time digesting and absorbing nutrients, regulating blood sugar levels, and providing accurate signals of satiety to the brain. **The best course of action for a healthy gut is to take a probiotic supplement daily**.

Probiotics are *live* bacteria found in fermented foods and supplements that promote gastrointestinal health. Probiotics assist in the breaking down of food and absorption of nutrients, which helps to reduce the production of gas and bloating.

For a healthy gut, it is critical to concentrate on including fermented foods in your diet like yogurt or kefir, pickles, and olives, as well as foods rich in omega-3 like fish, hemp, and walnuts. My favorite is drinking kombucha daily for my prebiotic and probiotic needs.

Prebiotics are a type of dietary fibers that the good bacteria in your digestive system "feed on."

Prebiotics are found naturally in:

- Beans
- Legumes
- Oats
- Berries
- Bananas

- Leeks

- Garlic

- Onions

- Artichokes

- Asparagus

- Nuts

- Leafy greens

Maintaining a healthy gut flora is essential for good metabolism and weight management. It is also very important for our mental health, as our gut health directly affects our mood. Dopamine and serotonin, the feel-good chemicals in the body, are produced and regulated in the gut.

If your gut health is poor, then your body will be less capable of converting amino acids from your food into neurotransmitters in your brain, and your emotional health will suffer.

Eat probiotic rich foods like:

- Pickles

- Feta cheese

- Olives

- Yogurt (contains live probiotics)

- Tzatziki

- Miso soup

- Kombucha

- Kefir (a fermented probiotic drink)

- Cottage cheese

- Sourdough bread

- Pickled vegetables

- Sauerkraut (fermented cabbage)

- Kimchi/Tempeh (fermented soybean)

- Labneh (fermented type of thick cheese yogurt)

- Any type of fermented food

#4: Boost Your Estrogen and Collagen Rich Foods

Phytoestrogens are a form of dietary estrogens that we get in our food. These are a plant-based nutrient that can enhance the hormone's health benefits naturally.

Studies show that phytoestrogens can reduce some menopausal symptoms, including the frequency of hot flashes and vaginal dryness.

The following foods contain phytoestrogens:

- Flaxseeds

- Soy products (tempeh, soy milk, tofu)

- Edamame

- Chocolate

- Legumes (beans, chickpeas, lentils, peanuts)

- Sesame seeds

- Nuts (cashews, almonds, pistachios)

- Garlic

- Fruit (peaches, nectarines, blueberries, strawberries)

- Cruciferous vegetables (broccoli, Brussels sprouts, kale)

Load Up on High-Collagen Foods

Collagen is a fiber-like structure in our body that plays a key role in **building** and **maintaining our bone and connective tissues**. It acts as the "glue" that holds the cells together, building and maintaining skin, muscles, cartilage, tendons and blood vessels. As we increase in age, we decrease in the natural production of collagen. This was my biggest side-effect of menopause: achy muscles and joints.

Symptoms of low collagen include:

- Achy joints
- Stiffness
- Leaky gut
- IBS (digestive issues)
- Wrinkles
- Dry skin
- Cellulite
- Thinning hair

And here are some spices and foods to add to your diet to increase your collagen production:

- Turmeric
- Ginger
- Green tea
- Acai
- Fatty fish
- Avocados
- Walnuts
- Sweet potatoes

- Kale
- Garlic
- Lemon
- Bananas
- Salmon
- Tofu
- Chicken
- Eggs
- Parmesan
- Goat milk yogurt
- Almond milk
- Quinoa
- Black beans
- Almond butter
- Cocoa powder

I added a daily collagen supplement to my daily routine, and it instantly made my joint pain disappear. Talk to you doctor about whether a collagen supplement is right for you.

#5: Eat High Omega-3 Foods

Research shows that eating the right kind of fat, in the right quantities, can increase energy, speed up metabolism, and alleviate depression. **Essential fats suppress appetite and decrease cravings for junk food** by satisfying the body's need for fat. **They can also reduce emotional triggers related to overeating and elevate our mood**. They will also help you burn more calories and feel more capable of exercise.

The best sources of essential fatty acids are:

- Eggs

- Avocado

- Fish

- Nuts

- Seeds

- Olive oil

- Flax oil

- Hempseed oil

- Walnut oil

- Pumpkinseed oil

A strict diet that skimps on calories from fat will cause us to feel tired all the time, which is counterproductive to good health.

Linoleic fatty acids (omega-3) and linolenic fatty acids (omega-6) are required to sustain life. Since the body cannot make them, they must be found in the diet—another reason why extremely low-fat diets are *not* a good idea.

Essential fats perform the following functions:

- Omega-3 helps reduce hot flashes.

- Essential fatty acids decrease food cravings.

- Essential fats increase the efficient delivery of oxygen and nutrients to the tissues by increasing the flexibility of the red blood cell membranes and making the insides of arteries more slippery.

- Essential fatty acids increase the production of hemoglobin, which increases the amount of oxygen available to cells.

- Essential fats optimize thyroid, adrenal, and other glandular functions, leading to an improved metabolic rate.

In short, our goal is to concentrate on eating good fats and avoid eating bad fats. Good fats include monounsaturated fats, polyunsaturated fats, and omega 3 fats:

Monounsaturated fats. This type of fat helps lower LDL Cholesterol ("bad" cholesterol) in the blood. It can be found in nuts, seeds, olive oil and canola oil.

Polyunsaturated fats. This type of fat lowers total cholesterol and triglycerides. It can be found in safflower, sunflower, corn and soybean oil. Flaxseeds themselves are also a source of polyunsaturated fat that you can sprinkle on salads or eat in your food. My favorite way to eat flaxseeds is in my breakfast cereal.

Omega 3 fats. This is a type of polyunsaturated fat, which lowers cholesterol, triglycerides, blood pressure and reduces blood clotting. It is found in high concentrations in oily fish (such as salmon, herring and mackerel) or fish oil (tablets or oil). It can also be found in flaxseed, canola, and soybean oil.

By bad fats, we're typically referring to saturated fats and trans fats:

Saturated fats. These increase cholesterol levels and increases the risk of heart disease. It is found in animal products, palm kernel oil and coconut oil.

Trans fats. Trans fats result from taking oil and processing it to form a solid fat (through a process called hydrogenation). This type of fat acts like saturated fat. It is found on *tons* of product labels, but a few common offenders include margarine, shortening, baked goods and processed foods.

#6: Bulk Up on Fiber-Rich Foods

Fiber is an indigestible type of carbohydrate which adds bulk to your food and slows the absorption of carbohydrates into the bloodstream. Unlike carbohydrate molecules, fiber does not get broken down into sugar molecules and instead passes through the digestive system undigested, almost like a broom sweeping the area clean.

Studies show that people with high fiber diets tend to have lower body weights. Additional studies have shown that most Americans consume only *half* of the fiber they need in a day. Lack of adequate fiber in the diet affects gut health, often causing constipation and bloating.

The best sources of fiber are whole grains, fruits and vegetables (preferably fresh with the skin on), legumes, nuts and seeds. Sweet potatoes are great to eat if you're having any kind of tummy trouble—they are easy to digest and loaded with roughage and nutrients.

You can get more fiber in your diet from:

Fruits	Vegetables	Legumes	Grains	Nuts and Seeds
Berries	Carrots	Black beans	Brown rice	Flaxseed
Apples	Spinach	Kidney beans	Whole wheat	Sunflower seeds
Pears	Sweet potatoes	Garbanzo beans	Oats	
Bananas	Brussels sprouts	Chickpeas	Barley	Chia seeds
Oranges	Broccoli	Lentils	Quinoa	
Mangoes	Corn			Pumpkin seeds
Prunes	Cabbage			
Dates	Kale			Almonds
Figs	Cauliflower			
Avocados	Celery			
	Asparagus			
	Mushrooms			

#7: Increase Your Water Intake

We frequently misinterpret thirst for hunger. When we feel like we need to eat, it's often just a drink of water that your body needs. This is called **phantom hunger.** This phantom hunger causes unnecessary calorie consumption and potential weight gain.

The confusion happens in the hypothalamus, the part of the brain that regulates hunger and thirst. When dehydration sets in, wires get crossed in the brain, and the brain misreads the body's thirst signals as hunger. In addition, without adequate water intake, the body cannot metabolize (break down) stored fat or carbohydrates, and waste will build up in the body, causing fatigue, bloating, gas and weight gain.

Bloating adds *extra* unnecessary inches to the waist. Unfortunately, many of us walk around in this semi-dehydrated state, not even knowing it. And this mild dehydration is often masked as feelings of hunger.

37 percent of people mistake thirst for hunger because their thirst signals are weak. Lack of hydration threatens the body's very survival, causing it to store fluid in *every* cell. This is the reason we get swollen feet, legs, hands and puffy eyes.

Signs of dehydration include (but are not limited to):

- Dry mouth
- Bad breath
- Headache

- Sticky saliva

- Chapped lips

- Weakness and fatigue

- Muscle cramps

- Rapid heartbeat

- Infrequent need to urinate or dark urine

- Dry skin

Most people know that a dry mouth is a sign of dehydration, **but dry mouth is actually an advanced sign of dehydration.** Do not wait until you have a dry mouth to drink water! Stay hydrated throughout your day. Make it a habit to drink regularly.

Water is the most effective solution for bloating and fluid retention. Remember when your mom warned you "not to fill up on liquid before your meal?" That was so you would have room to eat your food, as fluids fills us up fast. Water takes up space in the stomach, causing your body to tell your brain to stop eating. **Not only is water a natural appetite suppressant but it also is important in metabolizing and burning fat.** If weight loss is your goal, drink a glass of water *before* your meal. This simple habit will encourage you to eat less food.

Drink 6–8 glasses minimum per day of water, preferably more, depending on how much you exercise and sweat. Remember that pop, juice, coffee and tea do *not* hydrate you effectively. If you can't stand the taste of plain water, try **adding slices of lemon, cucumber, strawberries or oranges. Not only does this add flavor, but it can help you absorb the water you consume.**

Water and Mental Health

Every system in the body is dependent on water, and the brain is no exception. The more hydrated you are, the better your body *and* mind will work.

The brain itself is comprised of about 75 percent water. Research has linked dehydration to anxiety and depression because mental health is driven by the brain's activity. If the brain is *not* functioning optimally, your mental health will suffer.

Serotonin, the feel-good neurotransmitter, is dependent on water for its production. Without adequate water, serotonin *cannot* be made, leaving us vulnerable to feelings of depression.

Research found that women who drank *less than* two glasses of water a day were at *significantly* greater risk for depression than those that drank five glasses or more a day.

Do you need any more reasons to stay hydrated?

Fill up a water bottle, carry it with you, and sip throughout the day. Add a squirt of lemon juice or a flavored multivitamin package if you need some encouragement.

Pay attention to the color of your urine, as this is a natural indicator of your hydration level. Pale urine typically means that you've been drinking enough. Dark yellow, smelly urine is usually a bad sign, but keep in mind that taking certain vitamins and supplements may affect the color.

#8: Up Your Magnesium Intake

Lack of sleep contributes to increased weight gain, slower metabolism and increased fat storage. **It also increases the hormone ghrelin, which stimulates appetite, causing you to eat more and gain weight.**

When we are sleep deprived, we make **poor food choices.** How many times have you reached for quick, convenient foods which are high fat, high sugar, refined, and loaded with chemicals when you were exhausted? Too little or poor sleep can also **decrease** the hormone leptin, which helps you feel full.

Poor sleep can also make you up to 10 times more likely to become depressed. The problem is that roughly 60 percent of menopausal women experience sleep difficulties during menopause. How can we counteract this reality?

Answer: magnesium!

Magnesium is known to help regulate sleep. Magnesium is a nutrient that the body **depends on** to stay healthy. Magnesium is not made in the body and must come from the food we eat. Magnesium regulates nerve and muscle functions, blood sugar levels, blood pressure, and sleep. It is important for a healthy immune system, stress management, heartbeat, and bone strength.

Symptoms of *low* magnesium include:

- Leg cramps
- Irritability

- Insomnia
- Heart palpitations
- Constipation
- Headaches
- Migraines
- Tingling in legs
- Numbness in hands
- Weakness
- Depression

Some magnesium-rich foods are:

- Fish, such as salmon and halibut
- Spinach
- Edamame
- Avocados
- Broccoli
- Cashews
- Almonds
- Bananas

- Oatmeal

- Beans

- Dark green leafy vegetables

- Tofu

- Seeds

- Whole grains

Adding a magnesium supplement to your diet is also a good idea. Talk to your doctor about what is best for you.

Remember that these problems require a holistic approach to find solutions. In addition to eating well, a few simple lifestyle changes can go a long way:

Work on creating a sleep routine, one that you can reasonably follow every night to calm yourself down before bed. Keep your room cool, dress light, and use light bedding.

Turn off electronic devices at least two hours before you go to sleep and keep them out of your bedroom. If you absolutely must stare at a screen before bed, use blue-light glasses (can be purchased for cheap) or the "night light" feature (found in most devices' settings) to filter out blue light.

Regular exercise can help you sleep better as well as helping with weight management.

A Few More Gems

Vitamin D

Vitamin D is the most widely recommended vitamin for menopausal women. Many people say that vitamin D acts more like a hormone than a vitamin during menopause because a vitamin D deficiency can cause many problems.

As women approach menopause, the **body's ability to make vitamin D is *reduced* and its deficiency is known to *affect* estrogen levels, causing many menopause-related symptoms such as weight gain, hot flashes, depression, brittle bones, and mood swings**.

Vitamin D deficiency is also known to affect testosterone levels, causing symptoms like fatigue, weight gain, hair loss, brittle hair, mood swings and more.

Sunlight is your main source of vitamin D; however, your skin becomes **less efficient** at making it as you age, and the use of sunscreen **blocks** its effects.

To prevent the bone loss that occurs during menopause, a diet rich in both vitamin D and calcium is important.

Aim to include foods like salmon, tuna, cod liver oil, milk, yogurt, cheese, tofu, beans, mushrooms, sardines, egg yolks, spinach and kale into your diet. Talk to your doctor about how much vitamin D supplementation you should be taking.

The Magic of Apple Cider Vinegar

Apple cider vinegar has amazing natural healing properties. It is a natural antioxidant, full of friendly bacteria and enzymes. It encourages the body to **flush out toxins, help digestion and reduce symptoms of bloating.** It has alkalizing properties that help the body **reduce menopausal symptoms like headaches, night sweats, and hot flashes**.

Apple cider vinegar contains magnesium, the mineral essential in bone health and relaxation, which also **helps reduce mood swings and depression.**

Apple cider vinegar also helps with weight loss, as it reduces sugar cravings by moderating blood sugar fluctuations.

I personally love apple cider vinegar gummies. You can also use 1–2 teaspoons of apple cider vinegar as a salad dressing.

Chapter Takeaways

#1: Boost Your Satiety

Your key to healthy weight management during menopause is satiety. **Eating high satiety foods will help you to feel full for longer and more satisfied with your meal,** decreasing your overall calories intake and potential for weight gain.

#2: Bulk Up on High Water Content Foods

Adding a handful of high-water content foods to your meal will fill you up faster without all the extra calories of other foods. Aim for adding yummy foods with 80–95 percent water content to your meals.

#3: The Skinny on Water

Water imports nutrients and exports waste, including fat, to and from the body. **You must drink more water to lose fat and stay healthy mentally and physically.** Water also keeps your skin looking plump and healthy and reduces the appearance of wrinkles, bloating and constipation.

#4: Load Up on Your Menopause-Fighting Nutrients

Increase the eight key nutrients mentioned in this chapter to reduce the side effects of menopause. Strive to increase natural sources of all these in your diet to balance your hormones and keep your body running effectively with minimal weight gain and side effects. Talk to your doctor about taking additional supplements as needed.

#5: Take Care of Your Gut

Your gut health is critical for both your physical health and emotional well-being during menopause. Stick to a healthy, balanced, high fiber diet and consume probiotics and prebiotics daily.

CHAPTER 5

INCORPORATE DAILY PELVIC FLOOR AND CORE EXERCISES

Did you know that a protruding belly does not necessarily mean that you are overweight? Sometimes it is simply due to our **weak transverse abdominal muscles** that are not doing their job of "holding us in."

Poor posture, having multiple pregnancies, obesity, heavy lifting, carrying twins, carrying a heavy baby, and becoming pregnant later in life, can all increase the likelihood of having **abdominal splitting**. In fact,

50 percent of women have abdominal separation from pregnancy, causing a pot-bellied appearance and abdominal pain.

Abdominal splitting is a "tenting" along the middle of the stomach that happens due to an increase in intra-abdominal pressure that exceeds the ability of the muscles to stay intact. The **rectus abdominis or six pack muscles,** which are a strap-like muscle that run from the ribs to the pubic bone, become separated. The right and left sides of the abdominal muscles split from either weight gain, heavy lifting or pregnancy, and cause a noticeable and painful groove or valley along the center of the abs. This stretching causes the abdominals to spread because the muscles are no longer capable of compressing the organs and tissue inside the abdominal cavity.

To rectify the problem, you need tailored exercises to target the tiny intricate muscles of your core— namely, **your corset and girdle muscles.**

Understanding Your Core

The core is the group of muscles around your spine and pelvis that support and protect your low back and pelvis while you move. These muscles include the diaphragm, the **transversus abdominals** (TA), the obliques, the anterior pelvic floor muscles, the psoas and the lumbar multifidus.

Typically, these core muscles should "fire" or "activate" before you even think about moving. For example, if you wanted to lift something off a table, your body should fire its core before you even move your arm. That way, there is stabilization first, and then you are safe to add movement.

In a healthy body, this happens automatically and subconsciously. When there is a breakdown **or the muscles weaken with age**, the body fires the core too late, or not at all.

During menopause, in addition to hormonal weight gain around the midsection, we also become disconnected from our core muscles. Many people do not know how to *engage* these intricate muscles, causing the bigger rectus abdominal muscles to take over.

Unfortunately, when the "6-pack" muscles take over, the intricate corset muscles are not strengthened, and a pot belly remains. So, ignore all of those people who tell you to do 100 or 500 crunches a day—this will *never* get you a flat stomach, because you are simply working the *wrong* muscles!

In fact, the simple exercise of pulling your abdominal muscles inward, (upward if you can figure that out), and holding will give you more benefit than crunches when learning how to engage these important corset muscles. These are the muscles that are going to keep you pulled in and tight. **You must learn to activate your own corset muscles.**

Now just doing these exercises will not get you a flat stomach. If this is all you do, you will only achieve a corset activated under belly fat. If you want to have a slim waist, you must use **a combination of fat loss and strength training.**

How to Engage Your Corset Muscles

The innermost layer of abdominal wall muscle is called the **transversus abdominis (TA).**

The TA is the muscle that runs horizontally right around your body, from one side of your lumbar spine to the other. Lower down, it also runs from one hipbone to the other. Simply put, your **TA muscles pull your belly in**. They are a very important muscle to strengthen, learn how to engage and keep taught, as this is what gives you a **flat stomach**.

To isolate your TA muscles, try sneezing or coughing. Notice how your abs pull in when you sneeze, right? Those are your TA muscles working.

Try these exercises to engage your TA muscles:

Heel Walks

Heel walks encourage pelvic floor contraction while concentrating on the deep abdominal muscles as you walk your heels out and then back in.

Begin by lying on the floor with your heels bent, feet on the floor, toes pointing upwards. Draw your pelvic floor up, lock in your core, and walk or slide your heel away from you, slowly alternating your legs, and then back in again. It's important to only go out as far out as you can keep your back flat to the floor. You might need to build strength before you can walk or slide all the way out.

Note: The important point is to **keep the deep abdominal contraction the entire exercise, not releasing your pelvic floor muscles** as you move your legs. **To practice doing this, have someone put their hand** slightly under your lower back and make sure you are pressing down on their hand the entire exercise, not releasing until finished. If your lower back arches, or lifts off the floor, you have lost the deep contraction. Sounds easy, but it is not. This exercise is to be done slowly and controlled.

Draw in Your Abs and Hold

Simply stand and draw your navel in toward your spine (without moving your back or shoulders), hold for 15 seconds, and release. This can help you get rid of your lower ab pooch!

Abdominal Pull ups

Kneel with your hands and knees on the floor, back flat like a tabletop. Let your tummy dip down toward the floor as far as it will go (*without* moving your back). Then, using your abdominal muscles, pull your tummy up as high as it will go—imagine pulling your belly button in towards your spine, but make sure to keep your back still. Hold for 30 seconds, release, rest, and repeat. When you inhale, your belly and ribs should expand,

and when you exhale, your belly and ribs should contract and go up.

Breathe

Believe it or not, the best way to actually work the muscle that's going to give you your flat abs, is simply to *breathe* deeply. When you inhale, your diaphragm contracts and pushes down on your belly, which stimulates the TA to work. Inhale and hold the contraction for one minute.

So, if breathing is all we need for flat abs, why do most of us struggle with our bellies? The biggest challenge with working your TAs, is making sure that your other abdominal muscles are not taking over—a problem that most of us have, as our bodies naturally allow stronger muscles to compensate for the weaker ones.

Also, note that abdominal splitting hinders your ability to effectively isolate and "draw in" your oblique girdle muscles, giving you a smaller waistline appearance.

Posture and Bloating

Poor posture and bloating play a large role in our waistline and body appearance.

It's important to take good care of your digestion. **The best course of action for a healthy gut is to take a probiotic supplement daily.** Probiotics are live bacteria cultures found in certain foods and supplements that promote gastrointestinal health.

Another important element for a healthy body and good appearance is your posture. If you do not have good posture, you *cannot* have a flat stomach. The body mechanics do not work that way.

It's very easy to test your posture. Stand in front of a mirror and relax your arms by your sides. Once you're in position, look at your hands and see which direction your knuckles are facing (front, middle or back).

- If your knuckles are **all facing the front,** your chest is very tight and needs desperately to be stretched out and the back of your shoulders need to be strengthened.

- If your knuckles are **facing the back,** you must strengthen your chest and stretch out your back.

- If your knuckles are **facing the side,** you've got good posture.

Most people notice that their knuckles point between the side and front. The majority of us need to **stretch our chest muscles** and **strengthen the back of our shoulders and upper back to have good posture**.

You can stretch your chest by putting your lower arm (elbow, forearm, open hand) at 90-degree angle on the inside corner of a door frame), gently lean forward and twist away from your body.

Other great upper back exercises can be done with superman exercises of the upper, mid and lower shoulder area. My favorite is using the body ball, lying on it, tummy down, with the ball under your lower abdomen/hips:

- Gently balancing from your feet, raise your upper body off the ball (make sure you have your balance), place your hands out straight in front, beside your ears, thumbs up, shoulders down, and do 10–12 raises.

- Same as above but arms out to the sides, thumbs up, squeezing your shoulder blades together, do 10–12 raises.

- Same position as above, but arms beside your hips, pinky fingers up, shoulders rolled back and down, head in line with your spine, gently raise your arms up 10–12 times.

Good posture is critical for the appearance of a thin waistline, good body, and perkier breasts. Try it yourself; what happens to your stomach and overall body appearance when you hunch your shoulders forward?

Strengthen Your Pelvic Floor Muscles

The pelvic floor muscles are *crucial* to strengthen and cannot be ignored during menopause. Doing pelvic floor exercises will help reduce both urine and bowel incontinence—a *very* common occurrence during menopause. In fact, urinary incontinence affects over 50 percent of menopausal woman.

Every time you cough, sneeze, laugh, bend over, or pick something up, you will leak urine. Sometimes it's a little bit, other times it's a lot. For some, it's even full bladder leakage that will completely soak clothing.

There are two main types of urinary incontinence:

1. **Stress-related urinary incontinence.** When urine leaks out or squirts when you do simple things like cough, sneeze, laugh, bend over, or pick up a heavy object, like a bag of groceries. This is the most common type of urinary incontinence and affects 88 percent of those with urinary leakage.

2. **Urge incontinence.** This is when the **urge** to go to the bathroom is so sudden and strong that you don't get to the bathroom in time and lose control of your bladder.

Why does this happen? As we age, our muscles naturally weaken, and most people do *not* take the time to work on these very important intricate muscles to strengthen them back up again. To fight aging, weakened muscles, urinary incontinence and hemorrhoids, we must strengthen our pelvic floor muscles. No excuses!

Incontinence can happen with the bowels, too! For many women the urge to go to the bathroom is so quick and strong that they can't make it to the bathroom in time and soil themselves.

Strong pelvic floor muscles will not only will *prevent* **urine and bowel leakage, but they will** *improve* **your sex life and reduce constipation.** Unless you actively work on strengthening your pelvic floor muscles, your muscles will weaken, and urine leakage will happen. So, for all of you who don't want to take the time to work on these small muscles, you will be sorry!

The biggest challenge is learning how to "fire" these muscles correctly and on demand. You first need to find the **correct** muscles and then **connect** your brain to them. Most of us have a hard time connecting to these muscles and end up using other dominant muscles to "cheat."

What Are the Pelvic Floor Muscles?

Your pelvic floor muscles are the muscles that are tightly slung between your tailbone and your pubic bone, supporting your bowel, bladder, uterus and vagina. **You have front and back pelvic muscles: the "pee" and "fart" muscles. You should have separate control and strengthen both areas.**

To identify the "pee" muscles (or anterior pelvic floor muscles), imagine stopping the flow when you are peeing mid-stream, these are the muscles you want to engage.

To identify the "fart" muscles (or posterior pelvic floor muscles), imagine trying to stop a fart from coming out. These are the muscles you are wanting to engage.

The pee muscle is the area to target to stabilize your core and prevent urine leakage. The "fart" muscle will enhance sphincter control (the ring shape muscle of the anus), increase circulation, and reduce the risk of hemorrhoids.

Kegels 101

Kegels are a specific, **targeted** exercise that strengthens your pelvic floor area. Kegels should be performed **daily**–and there are no excuses for forgetting them, because you can do them anytime and anywhere, without others even noticing. You can even do them sitting in the car; I like to do mine when I'm stopped at a red light.

A little bit of effort goes a long way; you'll notice a big improvement very quickly. Once you've found how to engage your pelvic muscles correctly, you can strengthen them by doing **Kegel exercises, either sitting or standing.**

How to Do a Kegel Exercise

1. Draw **"in" and "up"** with your pee muscle as if to stop the flow of urine.
2. Contract **both** your pee and fart muscles together and then try and contract one without the other, alternating back and forth.
3. Perform quick, short and hard squeezes, holding for 5-10 seconds. Repeat 10 times.
4. Once you are comfortable with short contractions try and hold the contraction for longer durations. Hold up to 20 seconds, renewing the contraction if it fades.
5. Do *not* hold your breath.

Strong pelvic floor muscles will do the following:

- Increase bladder tone
- Reduce urinary incontinence
- Reduce bowel incontinence

- Tighten vaginal muscles, increasing sexual pleasure

- Reduce constipation

- Stop urine leakage when you cough, sneeze, bend or laugh

Other tips for practicing good bladder care include adding lots of fiber to your diet, as this will minimize constipation, which can put a lot of pressure on your bladder. Try to drain your bladder completely each time you go to the bathroom and sit down when you go to the bathroom to make sure you unload your bladder fully. Do *not* squat over the seat, as this will prevent you from unloading your bladder fully.

Chapter Takeaways

#1: Strengthen Your Core

Invest time and energy in strengthening your core to avoid many menopause-related symptoms, including urine leakage, hemorrhoids, vaginal loosening, lower back pain, and pelvic instability, bowel leakage, and protruding belly.

#2: Engage Your Corset and Girdle Muscles

Strengthening your transverse abdominals and oblique muscles will allow you to "pull in" your abs for a flatter stomach and smaller waistline, **countering the menopause-related thick waist syndrome.**

#3: Strengthen your Pelvic Floor Muscles

To prevent urinary and bowel incontinence and improve your sex life, make sure to **practice isolating and strengthening both your front and back pelvic floor muscles often.** A little prevention and strengthening will go a long way.

CHAPTER 6

NURTURE MINDFULNESS AND MINDFUL EATING

The practice of mindfulness is step #5 in the S.H.R.I.N.K. formula to critical good health and well-being during menopause.

When I first learned about mindfulness, I rolled my eyes, thinking that it meant only meditation and was not for me. But mindfulness is *so much more* than meditating or doing yoga (though there's nothing wrong with either one of them—both are great!).

Mindfulness is about being **present**, not focused on the past or the future. Mindfulness is about being **aware** of yourself and your surroundings. Mindfulness is about **accepting** where you are at currently, and not trying to change anything.

Mindfulness is about breathing, seeing, listening, and connecting to the present. Mindfulness is about experiencing one's own emotions and senses fully: touch, smell, sight, taste, and sound. Mindfulness is about participating in life and engaging in the now.

I know this may sound simple, but it is not. Most people spend the **majority** of their mental energy thinking, sometimes even obsessing, about the past or the future rather than engaging in the present. They put their energy into "wishing" and "wanting" something to be different in the future, or "longing" for something from the past.

Mindfulness is about committing to living in the present. You notice your experiences, and you **accept them unconditionally**. You pay attention to what is happening in and around you, without judgment, over-thinking, or invalidating your experiences. You avoid labelling things as "right," "wrong," "good" or "bad," "should" or "shouldn't."

To be healthy in body and mind, we *must* practice the art of mindfulness, and mindful eating.

Mindful Eating

Mindful eating involves paying 100 percent attention to the food you are eating *and* yourself around food. It is calm and peaceful eating, where you are aware of yourself, your emotions, and your hunger, and you eat accordingly.

Mindful eating is enjoying your food, taking the time to chew your food, and savouring every bite. Mindful eating is paying attention to the taste, flavor, texture of the food you are consuming and eating out of physical hunger. Mindful eating involves eating when you are hungry and stopping when you are full.

However, most of us eat without paying attention to what we are putting in our mouths. Have you ever finished the food on your plate and not realized that you ate it already?

Very often we eat fast and distractedly, shoving food in, not paying attention to what we are eating, almost like we are on autopilot. Then we go back for seconds or thirds because we are not satisfied and still hungry.

This mindless eating happens all the time and is a huge contributor to overeating and weight gain. We eat while watching TV, scrolling on our phones, standing at the fridge, or reading the newspaper.

Food often becomes more than food. It becomes a vehicle to satisfy our emotions; to numb, distract, hide, ignore, satisfy, excite. We eat when we are upset, sad, nervous, anxious, happy, frustrated, angry, and so on. Food becomes your lover, your best friend, your entertainment, your crutch.

It is critical to change the way we eat, and not eat based on cravings, desires or emotions during menopause. It's important to eat out of physical hunger, make wise food choices, and stay 100 percent present while eating.

Hunger

We must unlearn our old ways of eating before we can create healthy new ways of eating.

Let's begin by **defining hunger.** To manage your weight during menopause, it's critical to understand what TYPE of hunger you are experiencing.

There are two types of hunger: **physical and emotional.** The two hungers "start" in different places in the body, and the motivation to eat is very different. The only common denominator is food.

Emotional Hunger

Emotional hunger begins in the mind. **Although the hunger feels real, it is not.**

Emotional eating is when you eat in response to *feelings*—when you are sad, nervous, lonely, bored, upset or happy, rather than hungry. It is a "desire" or a "want" for food, usually after seeing, smelling, or *thinking* about a certain food.

Emotional eating typically involves eating non-nourishing convenience foods that are high in fat and carbohydrates. Emotional foods tend to be high in carbohydrates, as they allow more **L-tryptophan,** a mood-regulating amino acid, to enter the brain. Carbohydrates (and sugar) help the body to make **serotonin,** the "feel-good" neurotransmitter, so it makes sense why emotional eaters tend to consume foods that give them a "sugar high."

Emotional hunger can even determine the **temperature, texture, and taste** of the food we crave. When we feel **bored and lonely**, we often choose foods that are filling, warm, and comforting like mashed potatoes. When we're feeling **anxious or frustrated**, we often crave food that is crunchy and hard like potato chips. When we feel **sad**, we often want a favorite ice cream, pastry or fast food.

The problem with emotional eating is there is **no physical signal to stop eating, often causing overeating, overstuffing, and binging.** The emotional eater eats way beyond the point of feeling full, consuming unnecessary calories resulting in weight gain.

Physical Hunger

Unlike emotional hunger, **physical hunger is true hunger, and begins in the stomach**. This kind of hunger conveys a physiological need. The stomach feels empty; it may growl or give you hunger pangs. It even makes some people feel lightheaded or grouchy.

Physical hunger is a feedback mechanism that tells the body it needs fuel. The brain is the organ most sensitive to low blood-glucose levels. If physical hunger is not addressed, your blood glucose plummets, and, as a result, you may become irritated, tired, dizzy, or have trouble concentrating.

If you let yourself get to the point of becoming ravenously hungry, you are setting yourself up for overeating. When you wait too long to eat, you will often shove way too much food in your mouth to compensate for such hunger. You will become desperate for food and the hunger will overwhelm you. Avoid this destructive cycle by learning to recognize your body's hunger signals and eat *before* you get ravenous.

The reality is that most women do *not* even know what physical hunger feels like. **It is estimated that 75 percent of overeating is caused by emotions.** The best strategy is to aim to eat out of physical hunger 90 percent of the time.

Pre-menopause, my recommendation was 80 percent, but for menopause I've bumped that number up to 90 percent, because it is much harder to lose weight due to the slower metabolism.

Remember our goal is a lifestyle approach that you can continue for the rest of your life, *not* a restrictive eating program.

Avoid restricting foods, counting calories, measuring portions, starving yourself, depriving yourself of certain food groups, fasting for long periods of time or burning excessive amounts of calories. This does not work during menopause, and these are all *traps*! They may seem logical in the moment, but ultimately have the opposite effect for you, your body, and your metabolism by slowing you down, and depriving you of the joy of eating.

Identify When to Start and Stop Eating

A critical part of mindful eating is learning when you are hungry and when you are full. Using a simple **Hunger and Fullness Scale** (see page 121) will help you get in touch with your body's signals and re-learn when to start and stop eating.

When you feel physical hunger, ask yourself, "How hungry am I?" Rate your hunger on a scale of 0 to 10, where 0 is not hungry and 10 is ravenous.

Do the same thing when you are finished with your meal. "How full am I?" Rate your satiety on a scale of 0 to 10, where 0 is empty and 10 is stuffed.

Do this consistently for one week to heighten your awareness of your eating patterns.

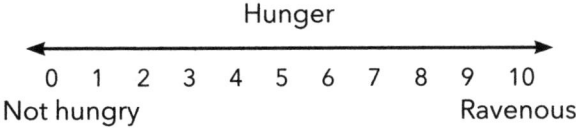

Hunger

0 1 2 3 4 5 6 7 8 9 10
Not hungry   Ravenous

Fullness

0 1 2 3 4 5 6 7 8 9 10
Empty   Stuffed

Practice starting to eat between the numbers 4–6 mark on the hunger scale and stopping around the 6–8 mark.

Many people have learned to eat to the point of stomach distension and pain. This is something to be unlearned, as stomach distension is a sign of overeating.

Over time, it is possible to learn to eat until you feel just right—not hungry, not stuffed, just pleasantly full.

Although satiety (fullness) signals are more difficult to recognize during menopause, they do *exist*, and you can become more attentive to them.

Your goal is to discover *when* your body needs proper nourishment and how *much* it needs. It may take a little time to relearn the feeling of hunger, so be patient; if you stick with it, you will learn to eat healthy portions naturally, without the fuss of calorie-counting or self-punishing compensations.

Focus on Nutritional Value

Just like gasoline comes in different grades, food comes in different qualities. By eating high quality whole foods, you increase your consumption of vitamins, minerals, and fiber, improving both your health and emotional well-being.

The best way to increase the **nutritional value (NV)** of your food is by getting back to the basics. Aim to eat more food that comes in its original form like fruits, vegetables, whole grains, beans, nuts, and seeds.

As a rule, the more processing and refining that is done to a product, the less nutritional value it has for you. For example, when grains are refined to make white flour, all that is left is a starch molecule, which acts as a simple carbohydrate (or sugar) in the body. Once in this form, the sugar is converted to glucose almost instantly, causing our blood sugar levels to spike high, then decrease quickly, often to a lower level than it was originally.

This causes us to need another fix of something sweet to keep us functioning and alert. Thus, the **sugar-addiction cycle continues**—up and down, high and low.

Processed foods not only lack nutrients vital to our health, but they contain large quantities of sugar, fat, salt, additives, and preservatives.

Sugar is in almost all processed foods, from cereals to flavoured yogurts to soups. Cells obtain energy from glucose or convert it to fat for long-term storage.

Food manufacturers often mask sugar on the ingredients list, making it hard to see the true sugar content of the food. For example, **you may see sugar listed as barley malt, fructose, corn syrup, lactose, rice syrup, ethyl maltol, or fruit juice concentrate**.

Scientific research indicates that a diet high in refined foods also *depletes* the body of vitamin B, causing fatigue and depression. Simple carbohydrates (sugars) have been shown to contribute to everything from obesity and depression to osteoporosis and impaired immunity.

If you have a choice between a muffin and coffee or a hearty bowl of oatmeal with yogurt and fresh fruit, choose the more natural one: oatmeal.

The goal is to eat foods in their original form as much as possible. Stay away from processed, refined, boxed food.

Here are a few easy substitutes you can make in your pantry right away:

- Brown rice instead of white rice

- Whole grain bread instead of white bagels

- A baked potato instead of French fries

- An apple instead of concentrated apple juice

- Cooked oatmeal instead of sugared boxed cereal

- Whole grain pasta instead of white pasta

Eat Protein with Meals

One of the easiest ways to boost your metabolism is **adding protein to every meal and snack.**

Protein produces the highest thermic effect from food and increases your metabolic rate by 30 percent. Thermic effect is the amount of energy it takes to digest, absorb and utilize a particular food. In other words, your body takes **more time** to digest protein than fat or carbs, so you **feel full for longer.**

Protein also adds satiety to meals, which will help reduce overeating. Focus on adding good quality protein like chicken breast, salmon, turkey, tofu, beans, lentils, eggs, or lower-fat dairy products to your meals and snacks.

Try simple things like adding a hard-boiled egg or roasted chicken to a salad, chicken to a stir-fry, and whey or low-fat yogurt to a smoothie. For a snack, grab an apple and a piece of low-fat cheese, celery and reduced-fat cream cheese, or low-fat cottage cheese and banana. Drinking protein shakes is another great strategy to keep you feeling full for longer.

Note: It's a good idea to eat protein before exercising to avoid using sugar stores as fuel. Try to avoid eating carbs 60 mins before your workout, as this will encourage your body to use fat as a main fuel instead of carbohydrates.

When carbohydrates are consumed pre-workout, your body will release insulin, which supresses the enzyme lipase for fat burning, and uses stored glycogen (sugar) for energy for your workout. This means that you'll use your body's sugar stores rather than fat stores for energy during your workout.

Eat Small Meals

The secret trick to healthy weight management is giving **your body less food to eat per sitting.**

It's a little bit of a mind game, especially since you might have to undo years of old patterns. But the reality is that many of us eat way more than we need per meal. Your body is dependent on fuel to function well, but it probably needs less than you think. By giving it small bursts of healthy, nutritious food, and not overwhelming it with things that are difficult to digest or too much food to process in one sitting, you'll be on a path to excellent weight management.

Years back, I was working with a 250-pound body-builder. I'll never forget how this huge guy would cut all his food in half and eat only one half now and the other half later to avoid overloading his system.

Eating small meals and spacing food consumption out throughout the day is key to successful weight management and less body fat storage.

Chew Your Food

One main concept of mindful eating is **chewing your food well**. Chewing your food is not only important for mindfulness, but also critical for swallowing, digestion, absorption of nutrients, and weight management.

Breaking food into small pieces allows the alpha-amylase enzyme in the saliva to begin its work of digesting food. **Ideally, you should chew each mouthful of food around 10–20 times.** When you eat too quickly, you do not digest your food properly. When you do not chew your food properly, large pieces will enter the digestive tracts and cause problems like gas, bloating, constipation, headaches and low energy.

Chewing breaks food down so that the body can extract nutrients efficiently and maximize flavor, increasing meal satisfaction and lowering the chance of overeating.

Chew your food, swish it around in your mouth. Ask yourself how it feels, what it tastes like. When saliva begins to break the food down in your mouth, the tastebuds on your tongue and roof of your mouth sense how your food tastes, and then sends taste signals to the brain. We have 5 taste senses: sweet, salty, sour, bitter, savory.

Even the simple act of smelling your food will activate the salivary glands, initiating digestion and getting the stomach ready for food.

Notice how food tastes going in your mouth; pay attention to the texture and temperature. Simply by slowing down and chewing more thoroughly, you will absorb more nutrients from your food, making you feel more satisfied and less likely to overeat.

Eat Calmly

Mindful eating involves **eating calmly**, savouring your food, and giving your brain time to catch up to your stomach. If you eat when you are stressed, the ability to digest your food will be **decreased dramatically** because your saliva production will slow down, and blood will be diverted *away* from your digestive system as part of the fight-or-flight response. You will end up **eating more** and **feeling less satisfied, with a sore stomach and digestive troubles.**

To create a healthy relationship with food, it is important to eat in a calm, relaxed manner.

Here are some quick tips to help:

- **If you don't already have a suitable place, create a peaceful, clutter-free eating environment.** Do not eat at your desk, at a table stacked with papers and books, or in your car.

- **Avoid distractions while you are eating.** Put down your book and turn off your phone, computer, or television.

- **Pay attention to what you are putting in your mouth, one mouthful at a time.** Even between bites, take a break, put your fork down, and relax.

- **Avoid snacking at the refrigerator or while preparing a meal.** It's easy to consume many extra unneeded calories this way.

Eat Warm Food

Focus on eating warm foods. **Warm foods are easier to taste and smell than cold foods and will increase your** *satiety*. Warm food is also easier to digest.

People who have weak digestion would do well to eat little-to-no raw or cold food or drinks. This means favoring cooked vegetables and fruits over raw ones, and choosing hot soups, stir-fries, or grain and bean dishes in place of sandwiches or snack-type meals. Freshly cooked foods are the most nourishing and free of molds or staleness.

Avoid Late Night Eating

We've all heard the importance of breaking the habit of late-night eating, but it is it's even *more* important during menopause.

Why? Because **food is fuel**. We need to eat food when we our bodies need fuel.

At the end of the day, most of our "work" is already done. It is *not* the time to load up on lots of calories. What ultimately happens is we consume more calories than the body needs, so the "extra" becomes stored energy, otherwise known as fat. The problem is we just keep eating more than we need each time, so we get an accumulation of "extra" energy storage that never gets used. This is how weight gain happens.

I know that it can be hard to find time and energy to eat properly during the day. However, it's important to aim to eat throughout the day and have dinner at a reasonable time—**ideally 3–4 hours before bedtime.**

Make sure to include some **good quality protein** with your meal, so you stay full and satiated.

Snacking in the evening is a mind game, not a body game. Your body is *not* hungry after your dinner, it is the mind that "wants" something.

If you've had a good well-balanced meal and you still find yourself hungry in the evening, choose something healthy with low calories like a yogurt or frozen grapes. Avoid doing this regularly, it is more about changing the habit and kicking emotional eating, than being physically hungry.

Change of any kind *will* feel uncomfortable at the beginning, including breaking the habit of eating late at night. But trust me, it is a habit you just need to break. Once you get past the difficult adjustment period, it will be smooth sailing from there, and you'll notice a big difference, in your body, mind and spirit. And then you'll look back and wonder why you emotionally ate in the first place.

Establish Regular Mealtimes

Having a similar mealtime every day is a good habit to form. This will allow you to plan ahead and be prepared, making it much easier to avoid binges, unnecessary calorie consumption and weight gain.

Make sure to pay attention to **how hungry** you feel when you eat to gauge **how much to eat**. Some days you may feel hungrier than others, depending on if you've had more activity or exercised that day.

When we were younger, many of us were encouraged to finish the food on our plate no matter what.

It is a much healthier idea to focus on **how hungry you feel** and **eat according to your hunger**, rather than eat according to what's on your plate.

Avoid finishing everything on your plate just because it is there in front of you. If you put too much on your plate, simply save it for later, ask for a to-go box, or just throw it out. There's no need to feel guilty about "wasting" a little food in order to take care of your body and mind.

If you let yourself get to the point of becoming ravenous, you are setting yourself up for overeating. When you wait too long to eat, you will often shove way too much food in your mouth to compensate for such hunger. You will become desperate for food and the hunger will overwhelm you. Avoid this destructive cycle by learning to recognize your body's hunger signals. Eat *before* you get ravenous.

Chapter Takeaways

#1: Practice Mindful Eating

Mindfulness is the key to a healthy, balanced life. Mindful eating is the key to a healthy body weight during menopause. **Mindful eating involves slowing down, being 100 percent present while eating, paying attention to every bite and chewing your food well.** Mindful eating is the opposite of mindless, emotional, automatic, stressed and binge eating. Remember, digestion begins in the mouth and eating mindfully decreases both overeating and weight gain.

#2: Re-Discover Physical Hunger

The majority of menopausal women have disconnected from their physical hunger, and eat too much causing extra calorie consumption, and unnecessary weight gain. **Aim to eat out of physical hunger 95 percent of the time.** Building a healthy relationship with food is critical in maintaining long-term health and weight management.

#3: Avoid Emotional Eating

It is important to undo our emotional connection with food, and avoid eating to numb, excite, distract, or fill an emotional void. **Although emotional eating feels great in the moment, it is a trap, and will lead to negative self-esteem, poor body image and excess body weight.** Avoid emotional eating 95 percent of the time. You can still enjoy food and "treat" yourself 5 percent of the time.

#4: Add Protein to Every Meal

Eating protein with your meals will help you to feel full for longer. Adding a small portion of protein to your meals will help you manage your hunger, prevent overeating, reduce food cravings, and help with overall weight management. It will also help to boost your metabolism.

#5: Eat Mini-Meals Throughout the Day

Aim to eat the majority of your food when you are active during the day. Aim for smaller, more frequent meals. Apply the concept of half now, half later by splitting your meals eating half now and saving the rest for later. This will help you to avoid fat storage and weight gain by overwhelming the body with too many calories at one sitting. Mini meals (morning, afternoon, early evening) boost your energy throughout the day and increase your metabolism.

CHAPTER 7

KNOW YOUR FEMALE POWERS WITH CONFIDENCE

Welcome to the final step of the S.H.R.I.N.K. formula. You will soon realize that you are more than your thoughts, and that you have the *power* to re-train your thinking to outsmart your negative thoughts and get more of what you want out of life, as well as tackle the remaining menopause symptoms from a different angle so that you can look and feel much better.

Feelings aren't a choice; we feel what we feel. But **our thoughts and behavior are a choice,** and we can learn to take control of them.

We must learn to believe in ourselves, to believe that we are worth good things. To be proactive and get on top of our problems, not underneath them.

This new stage in life is empowering. This is the time for self-love and self-actualization, the time to celebrate your successes.

Ask Yourself

Ask yourself, what do you want to achieve in this new chapter of life? What change(s) do you want to make?

I personally made a major move in my life to be closer to family. I left everything I knew to make a better decision for the sake of my family for the next 40 years. It felt very scary, but incredibly empowering.

What would you like to do differently in your life? What change would you like to make? This is the time to do it! Do what you need to do to make yourself happy, healthy and empowered.

There is something very attractive and sexy about a woman who is confident, who knows what she wants, and who has the courage to go out and get it.

Awaken Your Inner Goddess

Celebrate your shape! Own it. love it. Feel your beauty! You may not have a 25-inch waist anymore, but you are gorgeous!

Take care of your appearance. I personally believe in **dressing to flatter your figure. Accentuate your assets,** your good points.

Remember your metabolic body type; what are your best features? You definitely have some, even if you start with just your eyelashes!

For example, my best features are my shoulders and chest. I might wear a flattering V-cut or off-the-shoulder top to flatter my appearance and feel good about the way I look.

Make a list of what things you love about yourself:

1.

2.

3.

4.

5.

6.

7.

8.

The goal is to turn this stereotypically "negative and challenging" mid-life transitional time into a period of **opportunity, growth, feeling sexy, and empowerment for *you*!**

By reframing your experiences in your mind, you can create a different reality. **Menopause is a rite of passage.** Now it's time to embrace the wisdom, power, and beauty of this stage. Do *not* let anybody tell you that you are "past your prime," or no longer desirable or needed.

When I was walking with my neighbour, a 55-year-old woman who just completed her 12 months without a period, she told me that "she felt invisible." That hit me hard. Nobody should feel invisible.

We all have so much value. But, in her mind, she believed that she was no longer attractive, that she was "old," "washed up," "shriveled up" —that she was invisible.

After our little talk, that woman lost 30 pounds, earned a black belt in Karate, and is walking around with her head held high, taking care of herself and her appearance.

She no longer feels invisible.

Menopause is a different chapter, but it is definitely *not* the end of your story. **Turn the negatives into positives and fight back…gracefully.**

Although it may be uncomfortable for some of us to read about or discuss certain sensitive topics that we once wouldn't have, we must talk about what is happening to our "private parts" during menopause. In these times of female empowerment and celebration of our bodies we must open up the conversations about topics around the vagina, sex, breasts, odors etc., that were once taboo to talk about.

The S.H.R.I.N.K. formula is a holistic approach to menopause that deals with *all* aspects of the female body and mind, and this is a safe place to read and learn more about what you can do if you are experiencing any of these symptoms. There is no need to feel any shame. These are all natural changes due to age, and there are various natural solutions. You do *not* have to suffer in silence.

The reality is these "private" matters are often very stressful and confusing for women and too-often-than-not, they feel too embarrassed to bring them up to discuss with their doctor or friend.

To address these "issues," I've discussed many of them here in this goddess chapter because you deserve to feel amazing. There is nothing "bad" about what is happening to you. There is no shame in addressing these "issues" or looking for solutions.

This book, and my role, is to help you push through *all* areas of menopause.

Changes to the Vagina

#1: Vaginal Dryness

Vaginal dryness happens naturally as estrogen decreases with age. If you need, don't hesitate to use a natural lubricant. This can make all the difference in the world. Be aware that the vaginal wall absorbs whatever is in the cream, so stay away from nasty chemicals.

#2: Vaginal Wall Thinning

Vaginal wall thinning is a type of atrophy that happens due to decreased estrogen, and it can make sex uncomfortable. The skin becomes thin and inflamed, increasing pain and bleeding. This problem can be solved by bringing more blood to the area. Having more sexual activity, either with a partner or by yourself, will increase blood flow to the area.

#3: Vaginal Shortening

Menopause can result a vaginal shortening and/or tightening at the entrance. Having more sexual activity, either with a partner or by yourself, will improve your vaginal health.

Don't despair—these three things can all be improved. As they say, "practice makes perfect." You *can* improve strength, lubrication and elasticity of the vagina.

Make sure to do the following:

- Kegels

- Sex or masturbation

- Apply natural moisture

- Use vibrators (which can improve vaginal tone and blood flow)

- Strengthen your core and pelvic floor muscles

Go with the motto "use it or lose it" to get or keep your vaginal health. Be prepared to throw old beliefs out the door. Many women that I've talked to say that their best sex was actually after menopause.

Stay positive. You do *not* have to "throw in the towel" for a healthy sex life, unless you want to. For those of you who are no longer interested in sex, that is okay, too.

Sex During Menopause

As estrogen levels decline during menopause, the vagina changes. The consistency is different. It becomes dryer and thinner, which can cause pain during penetration and sexual activity. Some women choose to lubricate with a water-based lubricant to avoid vaginal dryness, bleeding and pain.

Go slowly to remedy vaginal tightness. Spend more time on foreplay. Work with your partner. Communicate your needs and wants. It may take longer for you to feel aroused and reach orgasm, so be patient.

On another note, your vagina and bladder will become more prone to bacterial infections during menopause, so be aware to keep the area extra clean.

Be proud of your body and express your needs. Talk to your doctor if you need more help. There *are* different solutions available.

Vaginal Odor

Some women complain about changes in the smell and consistency of their vagina and become self-conscious. In perimenopause, your vagina is acidic, but after menopause, your vagina becomes more alkaline. While this is a normal part of menopause for many women, it can be stressful and concerning, not to mention embarrassing.

Make sure to take a probiotic daily, as they help balance the changing ecosystem. Wear cotton, breathable underwear and change your panties as much as needed to keep things clean and dry down there. Personally, I swapped out a hair tie for a G-string in my purse. I don't go anywhere without an extra pair of panties.

Also, wash the external area with a mild, chemical-free feminine solution. Make sure to stay well hydrated and limit your sugar intake. Too many sugary foods will cause an overgrowth of yeast in the body.

And do be aware that sometimes an off smell can indicate an infection. Talk to your doctor or gynecologist if you notice anything fishy or painful.

Other Physical Changes During Menopause

#1: Body Odor

In addition to changing vaginal odors, you may also notice a change in your overall body odor.

Pre-menopause, I never used to sweat or have body odor at all; now, all the sudden, I've had to go through several deodorants to find something that actually works to deal with the underarm odor. Sound familiar?

Increased testosterone and cortisol are the culprits to this body odor change.

Take more showers, wear deodorant, antiperspirant, or a body spray. It's also a good idea to carry natural body wipes, wear breathable cotton clothing, and dress in layers that you can take off, and bring backup.

A little note on the difference between deodorant and anti-perspirant. Deodorants simply mask the smell, whereas antiperspirants stop the sweat by blocking the sweat glands, also masking the odor. I prefer deodorants, but if sweating is an issue, both are deemed to be safe.

If you find your smell unusually strong, talk to your doctor.

#2: Tender Breasts

Changing hormone levels can cause breast tenderness or soreness commonly experienced during menopause. **You may also notice that the size,**

shape, consistency and or sagginess of your breasts also changes.

Weight gain and fat re-distribution around the upper body affect our breast size during menopause. Milk glands shut down and get replaced by fatty tissue. And due to the decrease in estrogen, breast ducts and glands shrink, causing the breasts to lose their firmness.

Building up your chest or pectoral muscles can help lift your breasts and make them perkier. **Focus on doing exercises like modified push-ups (from your knees), chest presses, or push-ups.** You can also use resistance bands for chest exercises. To further support your breast tissue, it's a good idea to wear a supportive bra (if you can handle it).

#3: Constipation

Decreasing estrogen levels during menopause causes the colon to slow down. This gives the fecal matter in the system time to dry and harden, making it much harder to expel. For others, the weakening of the pelvic floor makes it harder to coordinate getting the stool out. All factors lead to increased risk of constipation and hemorrhoids.

It's critical to stay hydrated, eat lots of fiber from fruits, vegetables and whole grains, and to take your menopause nutrients. Listen carefully to your body's signals to have to get to the bathroom, never delay, and always stay calm and relaxed.

Experts suggest an ergonomically correct position when you sit on the toilet to expel. This position involves raising your knees above your hips, letting your tummy hang over your thighs and relaxing your pelvic floor. They recommend using a stool or squatty potty to elevate your feet.

#4: Itchy Skin

Fine lines and wrinkles are not the only skin issues to show up during menopause. If you're experiencing menopause dryness, and itchy skin, you're not alone.

As we age, our skin becomes dry, thin and itchy due to hormone changes and decreased estrogen levels. **A decline in estrogen slows down your sebaceous gland production of oils that hydrate and protect the skin.** The decline in estrogen also reduces collagen production, making the skin weaker and less elastic.

As a result, you might notice your skin is drier, itchier and flakier than normal. Things that didn't bother your skin before may bother you now. You might find that certain fabrics bother you now. (I personally had to give up wearing bras and any fabric other than cotton against my skin.)

As a remedy, it's important to use a natural body moisturizer that absorbs nicely into your skin, as well as a good face cream and eye cream. Stay clear of sulfates, harsh chemicals and fragrances. **Remember, it is best to apply moisturizing cream to your skin within 3 minutes of getting out of the bath or shower to lock in the moisture.**

Also, make note that our skin is made up of 64 percent water, so it is critical to stay hydrated. Focus on drinking good quality water—alkaline is my favorite. It is also a good idea to increase the amount of high-water content foods in your diet as well as increase your EFAs (essential fatty acids) like salmon, olives, avocado and olive oil.

Another great idea is to use a humidifier in the winter to help keep the skin from getting too dry and itchy.

#5: Achy Joints

Have you noticed that your hips, wrists, knees and/or shoulders hurt?

For me, I felt like I had carpal tunnel syndrome. The pain was so bad I couldn't write, I had to wear a wrist brace, and then suddenly, the pain went to my shoulder. It took me a while to figure out what was going on. One day, it dawned on me that something else must be the cause of these strange aches. Thanks again to our changing estrogen levels, our muscles and joints will get a little achy from time to time during menopause.

Maintaining a healthy body weight is the best way to manage your musculoskeletal pain. Luckily, this is something that we're already working on. Regular movement and exercise are also a great way to keep the joints lubricated and the muscles around the joints strong and healthy. Focus on low-impact, even non-weight bearing exercises like cycling, riding a recumbent bike, swimming, aquacise, and deep-water jogging.

Reducing your inflammation is another excellent strategy which can be achieved by concentrating on eating anti-inflammatory foods and a diet rich in vegetables, fruits, herbs and spices likes cinnamon and turmeric, berries, avocado, broccoli, green leafy vegetables, green tea and olive oil. You can also try adding EFAs to your diet by increasing the amount of fish in your diet.

Keeping hydrated is also very important. **Drinking lots of good quality water is essential to keeping the joints feeling healthy.** You can try adding sliced fruit or a vitamin pack if you need some flavor.

Taking a good collagen supplement is also very helpful—it was a life saver for me!

Turmeric also worked wonders for me. I took peach and mango turmeric gummies, and the achiness went away instantly.

Talk to your doctor about what is the best solution for you.

#6: Arms and Upper Back Thickness

I can honestly say one morning I woke up and my arms and upper back looked different then they had the day before. I had always had a thin upper body and then suddenly my arms and upper back got thicker, with a lot looser skin!! For a split second I thought, "OMG, I can't wear a tank top anymore!" But luckily, I knew what I was doing and what I needed to do and quickly threw that thought out of my head.

If this sounds familiar, don't despair. There is a way to take action and tighten up the area so you can feel more confident in short sleeves. **Try adding some triceps push-ups, triceps dips, or triceps extensions.** It's a good idea to balance that out by doing bicep and shoulder exercises too to give your arms nice definition as well.

You can also add **functional exercises** that involves using the upper body. Some sports that train upper body strength include rowing, tennis, squash, racquetball, pickleball and/or boxing.

Reducing your overall body weight, which you *are* going to accomplish through the techniques in this book, will help you reduce your arms and upper back thickness.

#7: Glutes and Thighs

During menopause, your weight typically shifts from your lower body to your middle because of hormones. So, if your hips, butt and thighs were an "area of concern" for you in the past, they are likely not the "issue" right now.

To tone the body, it's important to build the large muscles of your body, especially your leg muscles (quadriceps, hamstrings, and gluteal muscles). This will also help you increase your BMR (resting metabolic rate). **Remember, the more muscle mass you have, the more efficiently your body will burn calories.**

Try exercises like stationary lunges, alternating lunges, walking lunges, v-squats (plies), and squats.

Embrace That Female Power

Now that you are in a different headspace, a more positive headspace about menopause, you will be proactive about finding solutions to any issues or problems that arise. Whether its menopause's heart palpitations, thinning hair, yeast or bladder infections, constipation and hemorrhoids or whatever else menopause throws at you, there is a way through.

Finding your female power is transformative, opening a path to deeper self-awareness, wisdom and resilience. Menopause clearly is not a disease or loss; it is a transition. A transition that you worked hard to get to, and with it comes a great deal of wisdom. And with wisdom comes change.

Wisdom changes us. You might find that with this newfound wisdom comes letting go of and eliminating things or people that don't feel right to you anymore or drag you down. You might find that certain things or people don't belong in your life anymore. And that's okay!

You will likely be more selective with your time and energy, spending more quality time around things that matter to you. This is called **soul-care**. This is the time to take care of what matters to you on a deep level.

You might even find that you start sharing your wisdom with others. This is your female power. **There is so much beauty in being wise and confident in your own skin.**

Focus on the positives, and the ultimate in self-care...**self-fullness**. Really take care of you. Consider this a time of self-discovery. You have the power within you to create a fantastic new chapter of life. Don't let any negative thoughts, opinions, or limiting beliefs hold you back. Simply let any negative thoughts, if they arise, roll off your back not giving them any attention.

Focus on your power, your wisdom, your greatness. Now, go paint the world pink!

CHAPTER TAKEAWAYS

#1: The Menopause Paradigm Shift

Feelings aren't a choice; we feel what we feel. **But our thoughts and behavior are a choice, and we can learn to take control of them and use them to our advantage.** We can turn menopause into a positive experience.

#2: Take Charge of Your "Private" Menopause Issues

Turn all those "private" menopause-related symptoms into solvable problems. Say goodbye to dry vaginal, painful sex, body odor, constipation and much more…there are solutions.

#3: Step Into Your Wisdom

With menopause comes a shift in focus—a shift in where you put your energy and who you choose to invest your time with. Don't feel bad or guilty about letting go of things or people around you who are negatively affecting you or bringing down. **This is the time to practice soul-care and self-fullness.** Embrace your female power!

CONCLUSION

As you can see, it is absolutely possible to master your menopause and accomplish a menopause *without* pounds. In these pages, I have given you the roadmap, loaded with lots of tools and techniques, to help you manage your menopause symptoms and get through this transitional time looking great and feeling fabulous.

Now is the time to let yourself SHINE: beauty, wisdom, and strength. You are the DESIGNER of your life. Re-define. Re-invent. Re-calibrate. It's up to you, not anyone else, to determine what this next chapter of your life is going to look like.

Learn how to work *with* your body, not against it. Avoid getting stuck in the carbohydrate trap, the late-night eating trap, the emotional eating trap. Most importantly, don't get stuck in the trap of thinking "I'm invisible" or "I'm not desirable."

Follow the S.H.R.I.N.K. formula and you will learn to master your menopause. Take care of your physical body. Take care of YOU because it makes YOU feel better.

We all have some good days and some not so good days, and that's okay. What we want to do is increase our resilience and our ability to tolerate change.

Remember, diamonds are made from pressure. Push yourself so that you can SHINE.

Menopause is a gift, not a curse.

This is the beginning of a new chapter, not the end.

This is a whole new sexy, not old.

You are radiant, not invisible.

Beauty comes from the inside.

Shine like a diamond.

You *are* worth it.

You are GORGEOUS!

Let's do it! I believe in you!

—Michelle

ABOUT THE AUTHOR

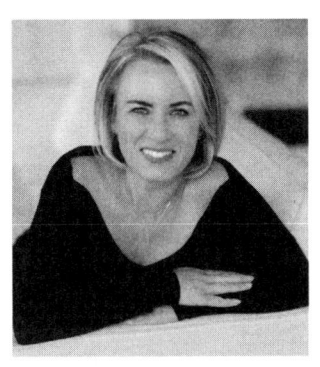

Michelle Biton is a leader and innovator in the health and wellness field. She has been inspiring women world-wide over the past 30 years through her books, newsletters and websites. Michelle is a health and wellness coach, mental health advocate and author of books *The Instant Anxiety Solution* and best-seller *Pregnancy Without Pounds*. Michelle is passionate about writing self-help books that empower people to change, implement healthy choices and live their best life possible.

Michelle has her master's degree in Holistic Nutrition, a bachelor's degree in psychology and a Certificate in Applied Science Health and Fitness Studies. Michelle has a background coaching people in mental health, addictions recovery, sensory integration disorder, behavioral coaching, disordered eating and anxiety.

Learn more at MichelleBiton.com.